The MIND Diet Plan and Cookbook

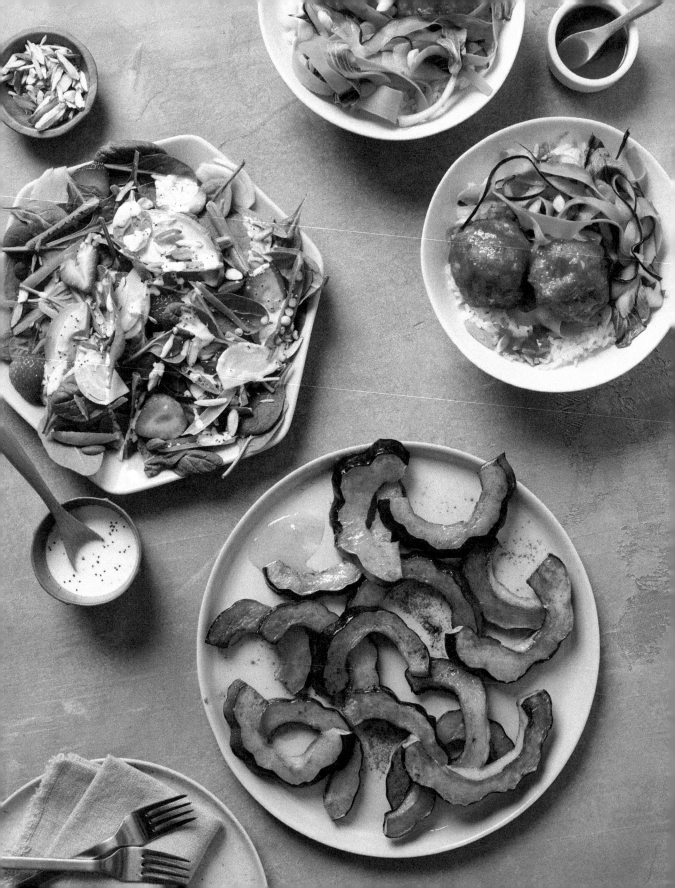

The
MIND Diet
Plan & Cookbook

Recipes and Lifestyle Guidelines to Help
Prevent Alzheimer's and Dementia

Julie Andrews, MS, RDN, CD

Photography by Evi Abeler

ROCKRIDGE
PRESS

Interior and Cover Designer: Merideth Harte
Photo Art Director: Sue Smith
Editor: Salwa Jabado
Production Editor: Andrew Yackira
Cover Photography © Nadine Greeff/Stocksy
Interior Photography © 2019 Evi Abeler. Food styling by Albane Sharrard.
Illustrations: © 2018 Charlie Layton, page 26

ISBN: Print 978-1-64152-442-1 | eBook 978-1-64152-443-8

Dear readers,

I never thought I'd have the opportunity to share my passion for cooking and balanced living with so many people, but I've learned to never stop reaching for the stars. I am humbled and honored to have authored this book and will cherish this experience for years to come. We will always be connected through our love of good food and our willingness to try new things in the name of good health, and for that I am forever grateful. Because of you, I have the best job in the entire world.

— Julie Andrews, MS, RDN, CD

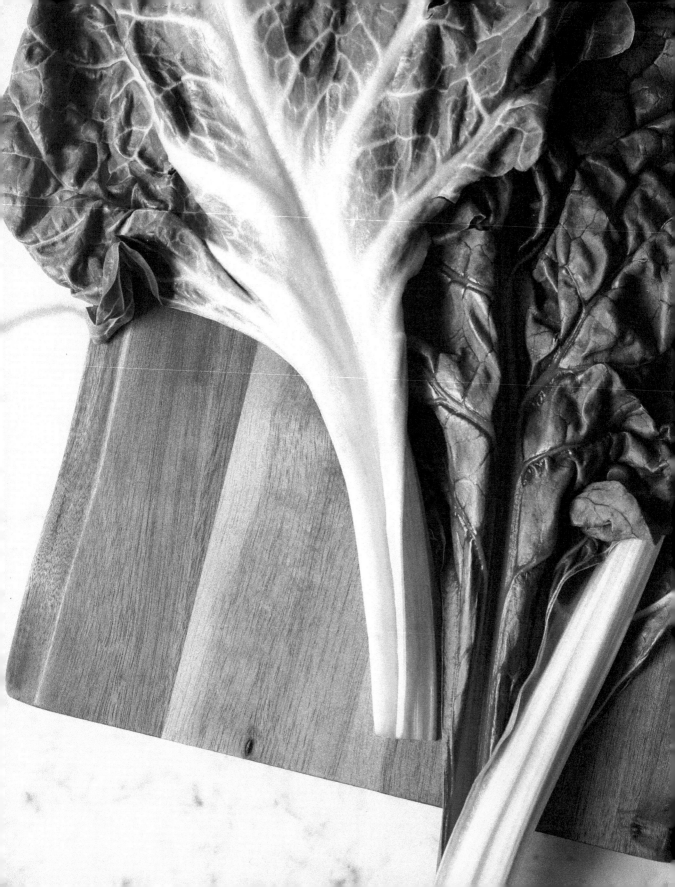

Contents

Introduction

YOU'VE LIKELY HEARD THE FAMOUS QUOTE BY HIPPOCRATES, "Let food be thy medicine and medicine be thy food." I wholeheartedly believe that food is medicine, from both a nutrition perspective and a nurturing perspective. Food serves as fuel for our bodies, providing us with energy and nutrients that can either preserve our health or hinder it. It's also a nurturer, as it speaks to our emotions, our cultures, and our personal histories. As a registered dietitian and chef, I am passionate about tying together the nutritional and nurturing aspects of food through cooking.

When it comes to nutrition, you're more likely to eat healthful foods when you prepare them yourself. Cooking can give you greater control over the nutrients you consume, and you can customize your diet to meet your health needs and goals. When it comes to health conditions—both preventing them and managing them—following a therapeutic diet and feeding yourself well can make a big difference, and learning to cook good food at home is a great way to set yourself up for success.

Cooking can also be therapeutic in an emotional sense: It can be satisfying to know that you crafted a meal for those you love as a way to care for them. There's nothing like the sense of pride that comes from taking simple, fresh ingredients and serving a dish that smells and tastes delicious. You create a deeper connection with the food you eat when you prepare it yourself. That sense of connection can help improve your relationship with food.

I have had the opportunity to see both the nutritional and nurturing aspects of cooking come to life. For several years, I led a teaching kitchen program for an academic medical center where I developed programs and taught patients how to cook for specific therapeutic diets. This included ketogenic cooking for epilepsy patients, low-FODMAP and gluten-free cooking for digestive health patients, and low-protein cooking for patients with phenylketonuria, better known as PKU—a life-threatening genetic condition that inhibits the metabolism of certain amino acids. I have also developed and taught cooking classes aimed at managing heart health, diabetes, and weight loss; preventing chronic conditions through improved nutrition; and offering general cooking guidance. I saw many people go from being intimidated in the kitchen (and quite frankly, annoyed by the idea of having to put a meal together every night for their families), to being confident with knife skills, simple cooking techniques, and meal planning. As a nutrition and food professional, there is nothing more satisfying

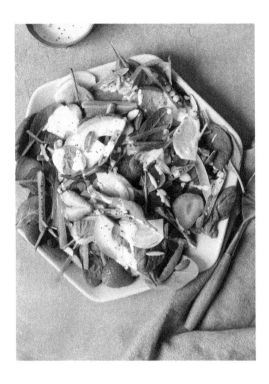
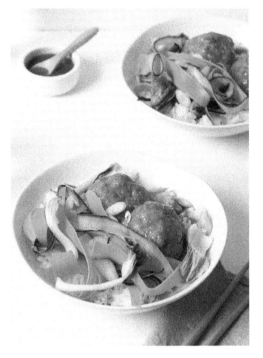

than seeing other people take care of their bodies and their health through cooking, and to see the positive changes manifest through improved health outcomes and improved quality of life.

Alzheimer's is a debilitating and devastating disease. Researchers have been working tirelessly to find cures and treatments, and research tells us that nutrition and lifestyle play a pivotal role in the prevention of cognitive decline. I am here to help you take the research and recommendations surrounding the MIND diet—a therapeutic diet for reducing your risk of Alzheimer's disease and dementia—and put them into practice in the kitchen. Just like I did with my patients in the teaching kitchen, I will show you how to cook and eat in a way that reduces your risk of Alzheimer's and dementia. I hope this book not only inspires you, but also shows you that food is a powerful tool for preserving the health of your brain and your entire body.

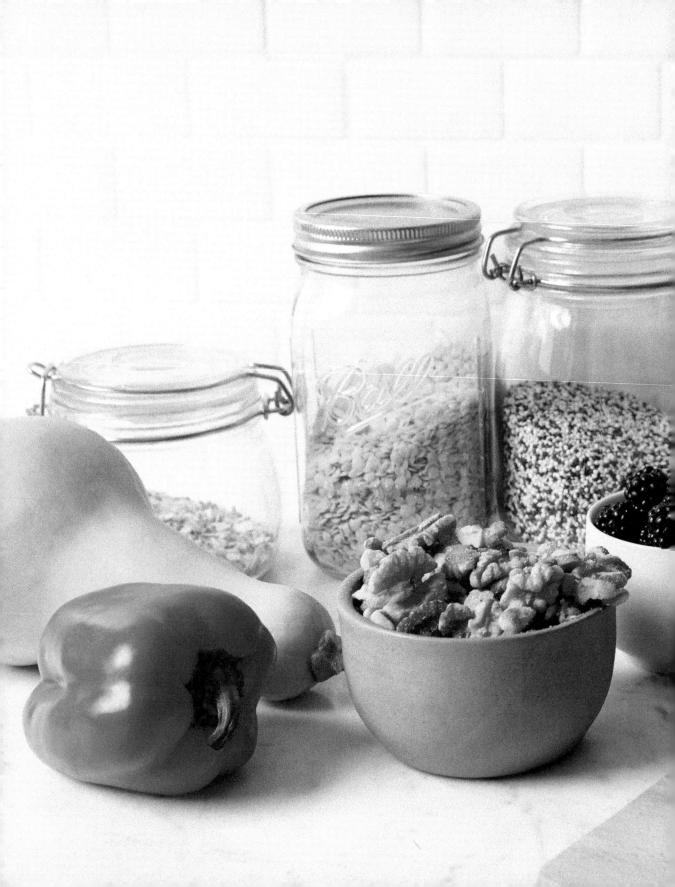

PART ONE

All About the MIND Diet and Meal Plan

The MIND diet is a set of therapeutic dietary recommendations, backed by research, that may help reduce your risk of developing Alzheimer's disease and dementia. This section contains an overview of the MIND diet, a list of recommended foods to include on a daily and weekly basis to improve your brain health, and a 28-day meal plan to help put the recommendations into practice in a delicious and simple way. The meal plan is also supplemented with shopping and prep lists, as well as a blank meal plan template so you can create one that fits your own lifestyle after the 28 days are over. My goal is to help you reduce your risk of Alzheimer's disease and dementia while simultaneously building your skills in the kitchen, growing your love for cooking, and improving your relationship with food.

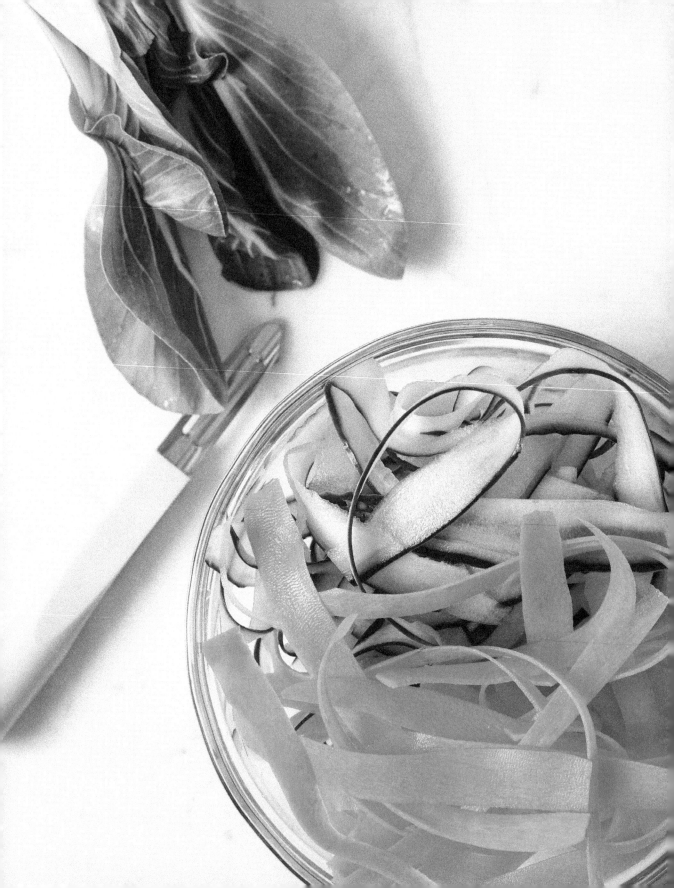

CHAPTER ONE

The MIND Diet

The research surrounding diet, lifestyle, and brain health is fascinating and promising. Because of studies conducted by researchers at Chicago's Rush University Medical Center, we now know that eating a certain way can either protect brain function or promote cognitive decline. The MIND diet is a set of nutritional recommendations that, if followed, can help preserve cognitive function and reduce your risk of developing Alzheimer's disease and dementia by up to 53 percent.

Dr. Martha Clare Morris, a nutritional epidemiologist and one of the leading researchers behind Rush University's MIND diet study, identified specific nutrients and foods that can help protect cognitive function when consumed on a daily and weekly basis, as well as other nutrients and foods that are associated with cognitive decline. In short, the MIND diet advocates for consuming foods rich in vitamins, heart-healthy fats, and phytochemicals that are found in seafood, poultry, and many plant foods, while reducing consumption of foods high in saturated and trans fats. I'll explain the principles of the diet in detail over the next few chapters.

A BRIEF OVERVIEW OF THE MIND DIET

MIND stands for Mediterranean-DASH Intervention for Neurodegenerative Delay, and as the acronym suggests, the MIND diet is a combination of two popular eating plans—the Mediterranean diet and the DASH diet.

The Mediterranean style of eating focuses on the consumption of omega-3-rich seafood, fruits and vegetables, whole grains, nuts and seeds, wine, and olive oil. While this style of eating has existed for a millennium and originated in the countries that border the Mediterranean Sea, it has become popular in the United States because it is linked to a lower risk of developing diseases prominent in Western culture, such as type 2 diabetes, some cancers, depression, stroke, and certain cardiovascular diseases.

The DASH (Dietary Approaches to Stop Hypertension) diet is a well-balanced eating plan that focuses on the consumption of potassium and fiber-rich foods while cutting back on sodium and saturated fat.

Both diets are rich in vegetables and fruits, whole grains, nuts and seeds, and vegetable oils, and are often recommended for people with heart conditions. The two diets are similar and complementary in many ways. Alzheimer's disease and dementia researchers took interest in these two diets because both have been proven to reduce blood pressure and are good for heart health, meaning they may also be good for the brain.

ALZHEIMER'S, DEMENTIA, AND COGNITIVE DECLINE

Although inherently different, Alzheimer's disease, dementia, and cognitive decline manifest in similar ways and can be difficult to differentiate.

- **Alzheimer's disease** is characterized by damaged nerve cells in the brain and is a type of dementia that causes problems with memory, thinking, and behavior.

- **Dementia** is not a disease, but a group of symptoms associated with a decline in memory severe enough to interfere with a person's daily activities.

- **Cognitive decline**, also known as mental decline or mild cognitive impairment, is a slip of memory that doesn't yet affect daily life.

As you can see, it's easy to confuse Alzheimer's disease, dementia, and cognitive decline, so I will address them each individually.

Alzheimer's Disease

Alzheimer's disease refers to a type of dementia that causes problems with memory, thinking, and behavior. According to the Alzheimer's Association, more than 5 million Americans are living with Alzheimer's disease and other forms of dementia. It's the sixth leading cause of death in the United States, and statistics show one in three older individuals die from Alzheimer's or dementia. It is an irreversible disease of the brain that progresses as time goes on. The National Institutes of Health characterizes the disease by the development of beta amyloid plaques and neurofibrillary tangles that cause a loss of connection between nerve cells and/or the death of nerve cells in the brain, which can block communication and disrupt normal functions and processes of the brain. Researchers believe that the plaque and tangle formations are caused by oxidation from harmful free radicals and inflammation. While some inflammation is a good thing, as it's how our bodies fight off infection, chronic inflammation is the root cause of many diseases.

In the early stages of Alzheimer's disease, someone may have slight loss of memory, but as it progresses, that person may lose the ability to carry on a conversation, pay attention, and remember newly learned information, and they may become easily confused and disoriented, have changes in mood and behavior, and lose their ability to swallow or perform normal movements or activities, like walking or using the bathroom.

The most common myth of Alzheimer's is that it's a disease of old age; this is untrue. Although age is a risk factor, the symptoms of Alzheimer's are not characteristic of aging.

While there is no cure for Alzheimer's disease, there are a variety of treatments that may help improve quality of life. The Alzheimer's Association suggests that early detection is crucial, as there are medications and lifestyle interventions that may help manage symptoms and preserve brain function, and individuals in the early stages of the disease may be eligible to participate in clinical trials.

Dementia

Dementia is a group of symptoms associated with a decline in mental abilities severe enough to interfere with a person's daily life and activities. Symptoms include loss of memory; communication and language changes; inability to focus, pay attention, reason, or judge; and changes in vision. Most cases of dementia are progressive, meaning that they start with mild symptoms such as losing common household items, and worsen to symptoms such as a decline in judgement, thinking, and reasoning skills. With dementia, brain cells are damaged, and depending on the type of cells and their function, symptoms will vary. Alzheimer's disease accounts for 60 to 80 percent of dementia cases. Vascular dementia, which occurs after having a stroke, is the second most common type of dementia.

In Alzheimer's disease, symptoms tend to start mildly and slowly progress to severe, while with vascular dementia, symptoms present abruptly.

Both Alzheimer's and dementia are diagnosed based on medical history, symptom review, physical examination, and lab tests. Like Alzheimer's, there is no cure for dementia, but some medications and treatments may help manage symptoms and improve quality of life. Diet and lifestyle can reduce your risk of developing dementia.

Cognitive Decline

Cognitive decline, also called mild cognitive impairment (MCI), is a slip of memory that doesn't affect (or only mildly affects) daily life. An individual with cognitive decline may forget things more often, such as appointments or events; have mild difficulty making decisions; have trouble finding their way around familiar places; show signs of poor judgement; or easily lose their train of thought. Symptoms of cognitive decline may worsen over time and increase the risk of developing Alzheimer's disease or other types of dementia. As people age, they naturally lose some of their cognitive function, but symptoms beyond a temporary slip of memory are of cause for concern. Following the MIND diet may preserve mental acuity.

Risk Factors for Alzheimer's, Dementia, and Cognitive Decline

Researchers long believed that genetics and age were the greatest risk factors for Alzheimer's and dementia, and that preventing the disease was somewhat out of our hands. These days, however, they've come a long way in finding prevention strategies related to diet, physical fitness, and lifestyle. One key aspect of Alzheimer's and dementia is their relationship with the cardiovascular system; because the heart feeds oxygen to other parts of the body, including the brain, cardiovascular health heavily impacts brain health. Some of the same strategies to protect the heart may also protect the brain, such as not smoking; maintaining normal levels of blood glucose, blood cholesterol, and blood pressure; maintaining a healthy weight; exercising regularly; and eating a well-balanced diet with key nutrients. Studies show that heart disease, type 2 diabetes, obesity, depression, and lack of participation in socially and mentally stimulating activities can increase your risk of Alzheimer's disease, dementia, and cognitive decline.

HOW DIET AFFECTS YOUR BRAIN

While it's no secret that following a balanced diet provides immense benefits for overall health, studies show that some specific macro- and micronutrients and some phytochemicals are linked to lowering the risk of developing Alzheimer's disease and dementia. According to the National Institutes of Health, key nutrients for preserving cognition include omega-3 fatty acids, vitamin E, B vitamins, and flavonoids. As we briefly discussed earlier, inflammation and oxidative stress are believed to be the cause of the hallmark plaques and tangles in Alzheimer's disease, and some of these nutrients are designed to minimize the damage caused by free radicals, which is why they're so important to consume on a regular basis.

Omega-3 Fatty Acids

Omega-3 fatty acids are polyunsaturated fats that have been associated with a reduced risk of many chronic conditions, both from dietary sources and supplementation. There are three types of omega-3 fatty acids: alpha linoleic acid (ALA), eicosatetraenoic acid (EPA), and docosahexaenoic acid (DHA). ALA is found in plant foods, such as canola oil, flax and chia seeds, and walnuts, and DHA and EPA are found in fatty fish such as salmon, trout, tuna, and mackerel. ALA is an essential nutrient, meaning the body cannot make it on its own, so it must be consumed in the diet. ALA can be converted to DHA and EPA in the body, but only in small amounts—therefore, it's recommended to eat both plant- and fish-based sources of omega-3s. DHA is of particular importance because it is the most abundant fat in the brain and helps carry out many of the organ's functions. As we get older, the levels of DHA decrease due to years of oxidative stress. Many studies, as outlined in a review in the journal *Nutrients*, show that DHA is protective against the development of Alzheimer's disease because of its role in membrane and neurotransmitter function and nerve conduction in the brain.

> *A 2003 study in* Archives of Neurology *showed that consuming just one serving of fatty fish per week was associated with a 60-percent reduction in the risk of Alzheimer's disease, compared to those who rarely or never eat fish.*

Vitamin E

Vitamin E is a fat-soluble vitamin found in abundance in nuts, seeds, green vegetables, some fortified grains and cereals, and plant-derived oils. A type of vitamin E called alpha-tocopherol is one of the few nutrients that has full access to the brain, meaning that it can travel to and from the brain to carry out antioxidant and anti-inflammatory tasks. Its main purpose is to attack free radicals and prevent damage to brain cells, also known as neurons. Researchers believe that vitamin E may also protect memory functions. A 2017 study in *Alzheimer's and Dementia* concluded that serum levels of alpha-tocopherol were significantly lower in study participants with Alzheimer's disease than in those who were cognitively intact.

B Vitamins

B vitamins are a water-soluble complex of eight micronutrients. Each vitamin is responsible for various functions in the body, such as metabolism, energy production, and cell division. While each has different functions, they require each other to carry out those tasks. B vitamins are of interest, particularly folate, vitamin B_6, and vitamin B_{12}, because they are required for the development and maintenance of brain function. Vitamin B_{12}, for example, is responsible for the synthesis of homocysteine; without this vitamin, the blood concentration of homocysteine increases and can cause cognitive impairment, according to a 2004 review in the *Journal of the Canadian Medical Association* and a 2007 study in *JAMA Neurology*. In the *JAMA Neurology* study, it was concluded that a higher intake of folate may reduce the risk of Alzheimer's disease.

Sources of folate include fruits, vegetables, whole grains, beans, and fortified breakfast cereals and grain products. Sources of vitamin B_6 include fortified breakfast cereals, beans, poultry, fish, dark leafy green vegetables, oranges, and cantaloupe. Sources of vitamin B_{12} include fish, poultry, red meat, eggs and dairy, and some fortified breakfast cereals.

Flavonoids

Flavonoids are natural compounds of phytochemicals found in plant foods that are beneficial to health in many ways because of their anti-inflammatory and antioxidant properties, according to a 2016 review in the *Journal of Nutritional Science*. While the mechanisms are unclear, researchers believe that flavonoids protect neurons from injury or death, suppress inflammation of the neurons, and may protect and promote memory, learning, and cognitive function, according to a study in *Genes & Nutrition*. Flavonoids may also help the vascular system work properly and promote new cell growth in a part of the brain called the hippocampus, which is responsible for memory. There are many subclasses of flavonoids, and some sources include berries, red wine, teas, cocoa, soybeans, legumes, and some fruits, vegetables, and herbs.

In the next chapter, we'll dig deeper into the foods and food groups recommended for preserving cognition and reducing the risk of Alzheimer's disease and dementia.

OTHER NUTRIENTS OF INTEREST

Research on two carotenoids, beta carotene (a precursor of vitamin A) and lutein, as they relate to brain health, is promising. Some studies show that consumption of beta carotene through food and/or supplementation has been linked to improved cognition. One study in *The Journal of Gerontology* showed that a higher plasma concentration of lutein was significantly associated with a decreased risk of all-cause dementia and Alzheimer's disease. Food sources of beta carotene and lutein include dark leafy green vegetables and red, orange, and yellow vegetables and fruits. A 2018 study in *Neurology* showed that consumption of 1 serving of green leafy vegetables per day may help slow cognitive decline associated with aging. Vitamin C is also a nutrient of interest because, although there is no conclusive evidence linking vitamin C directly to brain health, one of its main roles is to moderate and rebuild vitamin E, assuring it can carry out its function as an antioxidant and beyond.

A BRIEF OVERVIEW OF THE MEDITERRANEAN AND DASH DIETS

According to a 2013 study in the *American Journal of Clinical Nutrition*, high adherence to both the DASH and Mediterranean diets was associated with higher levels of cognitive function in elderly men and women over an 11-year period. This, among many other studies, sparked researchers' interest in how heart health and heart-healthy diets may be associated with reduced risks of Alzheimer's disease and dementia.

Mediterranean Diet

According to a 2016 review in *Frontiers in Nutrition*, risk factors for heart disease, stroke, type 2 diabetes, and other chronic diseases exacerbate age-associated cognitive decline, which can lead to Alzheimer's disease. There is also mounting evidence that the Mediterranean style of eating can reduce the risk of developing these conditions. According to a 2018 review in *Nutrition Today*, adopting the Mediterranean diet can reduce the risks of cardiovascular diseases, metabolic syndrome, obesity, type 2 diabetes, breast and other types of cancers, and Alzheimer's disease. As outlined by the Mayo Clinic, the Mediterranean diet's key components include eating primarily plant-based foods, such as vegetables, fruits, beans and legumes, whole grains, nuts, and seeds; using olive oil as the primary cooking oil, as well as other vegetable oils instead of butter or margarine; using herbs and spices instead of excessive salt when cooking; eating fish and poultry at least twice a week; and drinking red wine in moderation. Other key components of the Mediterranean diet are consuming meals with friends and family and adopting mindful eating habits, as well as exercising regularly.

Olive oil, particularly extra-virgin olive oil, is the main cooking fat in the Mediterranean diet. Not only is olive oil local to the diet's origin, but it contains monounsaturated fats (MUFAs), which are shown to help reduce LDL ("bad") cholesterol levels and increase HDL ("good") cholesterol levels in the blood. Fatty fish, which contains omega-3 fatty acids, is consumed at least two times a week, with some resources suggesting up to six servings a week on the Mediterranean diet. Some studies, according to the Mayo Clinic, show that moderate consumption of wine, particularly red, can reduce the risk of heart disease. Moderate consumption means no more than 5 ounces per day for women and no more than 10 ounces per day for men under the age of 65. Although there are no specific recommendations for total daily sodium consumption, it is recommended to season food mostly with herbs and spices, not only because they are salt-free, but because they often contain health-promoting compounds, such as antioxidants.

DASH Diet

The DASH diet is an eating plan that focuses on consuming a nutritious, well-balanced diet. While many diets focus on restricting certain foods and food groups, the DASH diet is all-inclusive. It places great emphasis on vegetables and fruits, whole grains, beans and legumes, nuts and seeds, lean meats, poultry and seafood, low-fat dairy, and heart-healthy oils, while limiting intake of saturated fat and sodium. Both the DASH and Mediterranean diets are consistently ranked as top diets on *U.S. News and World Report* because they are well-balanced, easy to follow, and have solid evidence to back up their efficacy in lowering blood pressure and supporting a healthy heart. As discussed, there is a strong link between cardiovascular health and brain health, and blood pressure is a key component of that. According to a study in *Frontiers in Nutrition*, increased blood pressure also increases the risk of stroke, neurodegeneration, and gray matter volume loss in the brain, which can result in cognitive dysfunction. High blood pressure is also often associated with high cholesterol, obesity, and type 2 diabetes, and researchers believe having these conditions may also increase risk of developing Alzheimer's disease and dementia. The hallmark 1997 DASH diet study in *The New England Journal of Medicine* showed that the DASH eating plan, rich in fruits, vegetables, and low-fat dairy products and low in saturated fats, can substantially lower blood pressure. A 2014 study in *Neurology* and a 2013 study in *The American Journal of Clinical Nutrition* concluded that adherence to DASH and Mediterranean diets were associated with higher levels of cognitive function and slower rates of cognitive decline.

Combining Mediterranean and DASH Diets into MIND

Research shows that both the Mediterranean and DASH diets are beneficial for cardiovascular health and can positively impact brain health, but the specific recommendations of the MIND diet are shown to have a greater impact on reducing one's risk of developing Alzheimer's disease and dementia than the Mediterranean and DASH diets alone.

> According to a MIND Diet study published in Alzheimer's and Dementia, *the estimated effect was a 53 percent reduction in Alzheimer's disease risk with high adherence to the MIND diet and a 35 percent reduction in risk with moderate adherence.*

By contrast, only those with the highest adherence to the Mediterranean and DASH diets had lower risks of developing Alzheimer's disease and dementia. All three diets are similar in that they recommend a mostly plant-based, whole-food diet with limited saturated fats, but the MIND diet recommends servings of foods like green leafy vegetables and berries because of the nutrients they contain and their impacts on cognitive function. The MIND diet also specifies daily and weekly consumption of nuts, beans and legumes, whole grains, poultry, olive oil, wine, and other vegetables, depending on the nutrient composition of the foods and their relationships with brain health.

As a registered dietitian, what I love most about the MIND diet is the modest recommendations for the consumption of specific "brain foods," which make the diet approachable and feasible. For example, foods like fish and berries, depending on your geographic location and the time of year, can be expensive, and consuming six servings of fatty fish per week, as outlined in some Mediterranean diet recommendations, may not be economically viable for many people, or simply may not be to everyone's taste. The MIND diet recommends one serving of fatty fish per week, which, to me, is a much more attainable goal.

In the MIND diet, there are a few foods of concern because they may contribute to cognitive decline if consumed in excess: red meats, butter, margarine, cheese, pastries/sweets, and fried/fast foods. Although some of these foods are considered whole, natural foods, such as red meats, butter, and cheese, they are high in saturated fat and should be limited to a few servings each week or less. Many people enjoy these foods, so it's my job as a registered dietitian to help patients and consumers incorporate them into their diet on a regular basis in a healthy way—after all, what good is a diet if no one wants to follow it?

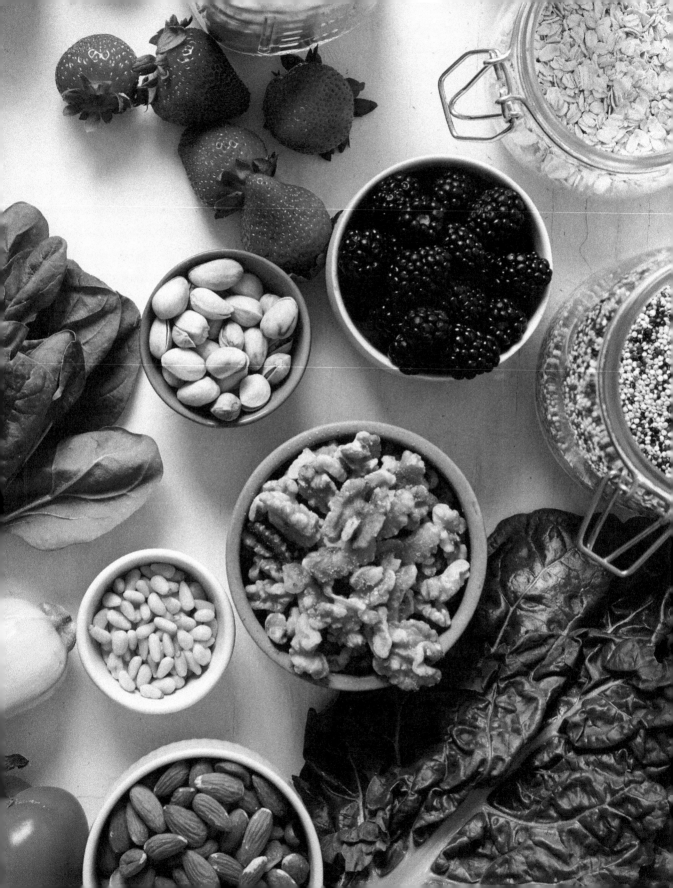

CHAPTER TWO

MIND Diet Recommendations

In chapter one, we discussed the MIND diet approach as a well-balanced eating plan that includes an abundance of nutrients to support cognitive function and brain health. Now, we will discuss what foods and food groups include brain-healthy nutrients and how often we should eat them to improve cognition and reduce the risk of developing Alzheimer's and dementia. Some foods and food groups should be consumed daily, while other foods and food groups can be consumed once or a few times a week. It is, of course, important to consider your favorite foods, your budget, seasonality, and what is feasible for you and your family when deciding what to cook and eat, but it's also important to consume MIND-friendly foods to reap the benefits.

HEALTHY MIND FOODS

MIND-friendly food groups include leafy greens, other vegetables, whole grains, berries, nuts, seafood, poultry, beans and legumes, and vegetable oils. While these are not the only foods you'll eat on the MIND diet, they should be the foods you consume most frequently, as they're loaded with nutrients. In the meal plan and recipe sections, I'll show you how to incorporate these foods into your favorite dishes.

Leafy Green Vegetables

Leafy green vegetables are perhaps the most important component of the MIND diet because they are rich in nutrients that are protective of cognition and brain function. These nutrients include vitamin E, folate, lutein, and beta carotene. Included in this food group are spinach, kale, mustard greens, Swiss and rainbow chard, turnip and beet greens, Napa cabbage, watercress, arugula, romaine lettuce, and spring mix. The 2012 Rush Memory Aging Project suggests that eating just one serving per day can make a significant impact on brain health. If you want to eat more than six servings per week, go for it! The more, the merrier. Here are a few simple tips to eat more leafy greens: Add spinach, kale, and mustard greens to smoothies, soups, stews, casseroles, and pasta dishes. Use spinach, kale, cabbage, arugula, romaine, and spring mix as the base of your salads.

Recommended number of servings: six or more per week
Serving size: 1 cup raw or ½ cup cooked

Other Vegetables

Vegetables are arguably the most important component of any healthy, balanced eating plan. They're loaded with fiber, vitamins, minerals, and antioxidants and are naturally low in calories and saturated fat. It's nearly impossible to overconsume vegetables, and most Americans don't consume enough of them. The MIND diet suggests that eating just one serving per day can provide immense benefits for brain health! While this is great news, I encourage you to eat vegetables with each meal. There are many ways to eat more veggies and to make them taste delicious. I like to roast vegetables until they're caramelized and crispy on the outside and tender on the inside (forget the days of soggy boiled Brussels sprouts!). I also like to add grated vegetables to baked goods and include a handful of them in my casseroles and soups. Shredded vegetables are also great in slaws and salads.

Recommended number of servings: at least one per day
Serving size: 1 cup raw or ½ cup cooked

Whole Grains and Starchy Vegetables

The MIND diet doesn't suggest avoiding carbs—it suggests that you enjoy the most fiber- and nutrient-dense versions of them. Whole grains are rich in B vitamins, are a moderate source of vitamin E, and are also rich in fiber and healthy fats. A grain is considered whole if all three parts (the bran, germ, and endosperm) are intact. Varieties of whole grains include brown rice, wheat, barley, wheat berries, kamut, farro, bulgur, corn, oats, rye, teff, spelt, and sorghum. Other good choices include quinoa, amaranth, millet, buckwheat, and wild rice. While the latter group are not technically grains, they have similar nutritional value and cooking properties to whole grains, so they are placed in the same category. When choosing products like breads, pastas, and crackers, opt for those that have "whole grains" as the first ingredient on the ingredient list or simply list the grain as the only ingredient. Also included in this category are potatoes, sweet potatoes, and winter squashes (such as butternut, acorn, and kabocha).

Recommended number of servings: three or more per day

Serving size: 1 slice whole-grain bread; ½ cup cooked brown rice, quinoa, or other grain; ½ cup cooked squash or corn; ½ cup cooked whole-grain pasta; 1 cup whole-grain cereal; 1 medium-size potato or sweet potato; 8-inch whole-grain tortilla; 3 cups cooked popcorn

Berries

While fruit of any sort is very nutritious, offering fiber, vitamins, minerals, and antioxidants, berries in particular are included in the MIND diet as a weekly food because of their flavonoid content. A 2012 experimental study published in *Annals of Neurology* concluded that a higher intake of berries, which contain flavonoids called anthocyanidins, appears to reduce rates of cognitive decline in older adults. In a 2018 study published in the *European Journal of Nutrition,* participants who consumed freeze-dried blueberries equivalent to 1 cup of blueberries per day showed significantly fewer repetition errors in learning tests in comparison to the control group. And in the Nurses' Health Study, those who consumed blueberries one or more times per week had slower rates of cognitive decline than those who consumed blueberries less than once per week. Berries are versatile—perfect as a topping for pancakes, waffles, yogurt, or oatmeal; frozen and added to smoothies; or as the featured ingredient in a leafy green salad. I also like to incorporate them into desserts, which you'll see in chapter nine (page 199).

Recommended number of servings: two or more per week
Serving size: ½ cup raw or frozen

A NOTE ON FRUIT

It is also important to note that when the MIND diet was written in 2015, there were no studies that linked fruit consumption, in general, to lowering the risk of cognitive decline. However, an observational study published in *Neurology* in 2018 concluded that higher intakes of total vegetables, total fruits, and fruit juice were significantly associated with lower odds of moderate or poor subjective cognitive function (SCF). SCF is a patient's report of their thinking abilities, including loss of memory, increasing forgetfulness, losing their train of thought, and feeling overwhelmed making decisions or planning, according to Cedars-Sinai. As mentioned earlier, all fruits—not just berries—are nutrient-dense, so it's important to consume a variety of them to support overall health.

PORTION CONTROL

Being aware of portion sizes for common foods can be helpful and eye-opening. Here are some portion-size guidelines to keep in mind:

FIST	**PALM**	**HANDFUL**	**THUMB**
1 cup	3–4 ounces	1 ounce	1 ounce or 1–2 tablespoons
Raw, non-starchy vegetables	Seafood Poultry	Nuts Seeds	Cheese Nut Butter

Nuts

It's no secret that nuts are loaded with nutrients, such as vitamin E, B vitamins, healthy fats, and a variety of minerals. Each nut offers a unique nutrient profile, but overall, we know they are good for brain health. In a 2014 observational study published in the *Journal of Nutrition, Health & Aging*, it was concluded that higher long-term total nut intake was associated with better cognition, and women who consumed at least five servings of nuts per week had higher cognitive scores than those who did not consume nuts. In a 2012 study published in the *Journal of Alzheimer's Disease*, researchers found that consumption of walnuts, specifically, was associated with better working memory scores; this could be because walnuts have the highest antioxidant capacity and are richest in omega-3 fatty acids, compared to other nuts. The MIND diet recommends consuming a variety of nuts, including walnuts, pecans, pistachios, almonds, cashews, macadamia nuts, Brazil nuts, and peanuts. They serve as a filling snack; provide crunch and flavor to salads, curries, and Asian dishes; and add texture to desserts.

Recommended number of servings: five or more per week
Serving size: 1 ounce

CONCERNS ABOUT MERCURY

There are trace levels of mercury in nearly every type of seafood. For most people, consuming seafood does not pose a health threat, but the FDA and EPA advise women who may become pregnant, pregnant women, nursing moms, and young children to avoid types of seafood that are high in mercury, such as bigeye tuna (not canned), mackerel, shark, tilefish, marlin, orange roughy, and swordfish.

Seafood

Seafood is one of the few food sources of DHA, the type of omega-3 that can protect the brain from the effects of oxidative stress. According to Seafood Health Facts, several types of seafood contain high amounts of omega-3 fatty acids, including salmon, herring, mackerel, tuna, sardines, rainbow trout, oysters, and mussels. Other types of seafood with moderate amounts of omega-3s include Alaskan pollock, rockfish, clams, crab, lobster, snapper, grouper, flounder, sole, halibut, ocean perch, and squid. There are small amounts of omega-3s in scallops, shrimp, cod, haddock, tilapia, catfish, mahi mahi, orange roughy, and imitation crab. MIND diet research shows that consuming just one serving of omega-3-rich seafood per week can positively impact brain health. And if you enjoy fish and shellfish, there is no harm in consuming it more than once a week. Also note that while wild-caught fish has the highest levels of omega-3s, farmed and canned varieties still provide a hefty dose. In chapter seven (page 139), you'll find a variety of seafood recipes.

Recommended number of servings: one or more per week
Serving size: 3 to 4 ounces

Poultry

Chicken and turkey are popular forms of protein in the American diet, as they taste mild, are relatively affordable, and are versatile to cook with. Lean varieties of poultry include the breast and wings, often referred to as white meat. Dark meat from the thighs and legs and the chicken skin are all high in saturated fat. That's not to say that you can't enjoy the thighs and legs, as they are quite tasty, but I recommend consuming the leaner cuts more often. Poultry is also a great source of B vitamins, which are linked to brain health. Cooked boneless, skinless chicken breasts can be used in salads, soups, casseroles, bowls, and tacos. Since they are lean, it helps to marinate them or rub them with spices, and to grill them, sauté them in olive oil, or roast them. No matter the cooking method, it's important to cook poultry properly so it does not become dry; your best bet is to use an instant-read thermometer and cook to 165°F.

Recommended number of servings: two or more per week
Serving size: 3 to 4 ounces

Beans and Legumes

Beans and legumes are an inexpensive way to load up your diet with B vitamins, protein, and fiber. It is great news that beans and legumes are loaded with nutrition, because they're inexpensive, easy to prepare, and can be incorporated into almost everything we eat—even dessert! There are many varieties of beans, including light and dark red kidneys, cannellinis, great northerns, pintos, black beans, and chickpeas (a.k.a. garbanzo beans). Other types of legumes include lentils, peas, lima beans, and soybeans, including edamame and tofu. The canned varieties of beans and legumes are most convenient, but if you're interested in prepping and cooking dried beans and legumes you can save some money, and you might even like the taste and texture a little better than canned. When choosing canned beans, opt for low-sodium or no-added-salt versions. It's wise to choose canned foods with little or no added salt so you're in control of how much sodium you consume in a finished meal.

Recommended number of servings: three or more per week
Serving size: ½ cup cooked

Vegetable Oils

There are seemingly endless oil options in the supermarket, each marketed as the best oil for your culinary needs. This can make it difficult to decide which oil to use, and when. The MIND diet recommends using extra-virgin olive oil because of its nutrient profile: It contains mostly monounsaturated fats, vitamin E, and antioxidants. However, the one downfall of extra-virgin olive oil is that it has a low smoke point, meaning it burns easily and should not be used for high-heat cooking, such as grilling and roasting. I use extra-virgin olive oil for medium-heat cooking, such as sautéing, and for making salad dressings and drizzling on finished dishes. I use other vegetable oils for high-heat cooking, such as avocado and canola oils. They both have high smoke points and are relatively healthy. Avocado oil is mostly made up of monounsaturated fats, which studies show can increase HDL ("good") cholesterol. Canola oil is rich in the omega-3 fatty acid ALA. I use nut oils for flavoring and finishing, especially when a particular oil's flavor pairs well with the dish I'm making. Other types of vegetable oils include corn, cottonseed, grapeseed, peanut, safflower, soybean, and sunflower. I do not typically cook with and do not recommend cooking with these oils, because we typically consume enough of them in processed foods and restaurant dishes; I only use avocado, canola, and extra-virgin olive oil when cooking at home.

Recommended number of servings: as needed for cooking and/or finishing dishes
Serving size: 1 tablespoon

Foods to Limit

While I'm not a fan of restriction, as I believe part of a healthy diet is having a good relationship with food and feeling free to consume the foods you love, it is important to note that some foods, when consumed in excess, can increase inflammation, raise blood pressure and blood glucose, and increase your risk of developing chronic conditions. That's why it's critical to understand what research tells us—especially as it relates to brain health—to develop a balanced plan so you can be successful in reaching your health goals *and* enjoy what you eat. (Yes, it is possible to do both!) The thing

WINE AND THE MIND DIET

A glass of wine a day keeps the doctor away? Sounds too good to be true, but studies show that consuming alcohol in moderation can protect your heart and your brain. In a 2012 review published in *Frontiers in Bioscience*, researchers concluded that those whose consumption of alcohol is light to moderate, as compared to those who never drink or excessively consume, have lower risks of age-dependent cognitive decline and dementia, including Alzheimer's disease. Numerous studies show that moderate wine consumption reduces cardiovascular and neurodegenerative mortality. Wine contains a compound called resveratrol that has antioxidant properties, which is the reason for the hype surrounding wine consumption and health. The MIND diet suggests consuming one 5-ounce glass of wine per day. If you're a non-drinker, that doesn't mean you have to start drinking to be healthy. Keep in mind that alcohol can be addictive, so those with a personal or family history of alcoholism should abstain. It's wise to discuss alcohol intake with your doctor.

ALL ABOUT FATS

When it comes to fats, it's recommended that you consume mono- and polyunsaturated fats most often, saturated fats sometimes, and trans fats very rarely (if at all).

The Dietary Guidelines for Americans suggests consuming no more than 10 percent of your calories from saturated fat. Trans fats, labeled as hydrogenated oils, are linked to cardiovascular diseases.

In *Archives of Neurology*, one 2003 study showed that the consumption of trans fatty acids may increase one's risk of Alzheimer's disease.

However, a 2011 study published in the *Journal of the American Geriatrics Society* showed no association between saturated and trans fat intake and cognitive decline, but did find that monounsaturated fats were associated with less cognitive decline. It's clear that more research needs to be done on saturated and trans fats and their relationships with brain health, but we do know that high intake of saturated and trans fats—especially trans fats—are linked to increased risks of cardiovasular diseases.

to remember is that small amounts of the foods I'm about to discuss will likely not increase your risks of cognitive decline or cardiovascular diseases, so feel free to enjoy them in moderation.

Red Meat

The concern with red meat surrounds its saturated fat content. The MIND diet suggests consuming no more than three servings of red meat per week. While there is no direct research that "blames" cognitive decline on the consumption of red meat, we do know that excessive saturated fat intake can increase your risk for cardiovascular diseases, which can impact brain function. Again, this does not mean you should cut out red meat entirely, but if you enjoy red meat daily, for example, I'd suggest swapping out one or two meals with seafood or poultry. When you do enjoy red meat dishes, choose cuts that are lean, such as tenderloin, sirloin, and top round. It is important to note that red meat is a great source of vitamin B_{12} and iron.

Recommended number of servings: three or less per week
Serving size: 3 ounces for women; 5 ounces for men

Whole-Fat Dairy Products

Butter, cream, and cheese are all delicious parts of the traditional American diet. Like red meat, these foods are high in saturated fat, so I suggest using small amounts to enhance a dish, rather than having them as the main ingredient. For example, sprinkle Parmesan or Cheddar cheese on casseroles or tacos to add a cheesy, salty flavor, or finish puréed soups with a few tablespoons of cream to add richness. And, of course, you may want to enjoy cookies or pastries made with real butter from time to time, and I suggest real butter instead of margarine because most margarines contain trans fats.

Recommended number of servings: one serving of butter per day; one serving or less of cheese per week
Serving size: 1 tablespoon butter; 1 ounce cheese

Fried Foods

Deep-fried foods like French fries, donuts, and fried chicken are high in trans and saturated fats. In addition, deep-fried foods typically do not provide much nutrition, in comparison to leafy greens, vegetables, fruits, whole grains, beans, legumes, poultry, and olive oil.

Recommended number of servings: one or less per week
Serving size: one donut; one small order of French fries

Sweets and Pastries

While there are no research studies that link dessert intake with cognitive decline, foods such as sweets and pastries are generally high in sugar and "bad" fats, and often don't provide much nutritional value. The MIND diet focuses more on consuming foods that are packed with brain-supportive nutrients. As I've previously mentioned, I believe it's important to include foods in your diet that are indulgent, but to be strategic about it. You should never feel deprived or restricted, and I've taken that to heart throughout this book. The MIND diet desserts I developed for this book are plenty indulgent, but each one also contains some MIND diet–friendly foods to keep you on track.

Recommended number of servings: less than five per week
Serving size: one cookie; one piece of cake or pie; one cupcake

MIND Diet Food Lists

Encourage	Limit	Avoid
Leafy green vegetables	Red meat (such as beef, pork, and lamb)	Trans fats (choose foods without hydrogenated oils)
Other vegetables	Whole-fat dairy	
Whole grains and starchy vegetables	Fried foods	
Berries	Sweets and pastries	
Nuts	Wine	
Seafood (such as salmon, tuna, and cod)		
Poultry (lean white meat)		
Beans and legumes		
Vegetable oils (such as olive oil and avocado oil)		

MIND DIET FOODS BY THE SEASONS

As the seasons come and go, so do fresh fruits and vegetables. The good news is that frozen fruits and vegetables are generally just as nutritious as fresh and are available year-round. Frozen produce is generally picked at peak ripeness and immediately frozen, so it does not lose nutrients during transport. Canned and dried fruits and vegetables are also nutritious, as long as they don't contain added ingredients like sugar and salt.

Spring

Apricots
Asparagus
Broccoli
Collard greens

Kale
Kiwifruit
Lettuce
Mushrooms

Onions
Peas
Radishes
Rhubarb

Spinach
Strawberries
Swiss chard
Turnips

Summer

Beets
Bell peppers
Blackberries
Blueberries
Cantaloupe
Cherries

Corn
Cucumbers
Eggplant
Green beans
Honeydew melon
Lima beans

Mangoes
Okra
Peaches
Plums
Raspberries
Strawberries

Summer squash
Tomatillos
Tomatoes
Watermelon
Wax beans
Zucchini

Fall

Beets
Bell peppers
Broccoli
Brussels sprouts
Cabbage
Cauliflower
Collard greens
Cranberries

Ginger
Grapes
Green beans
Kale
Kiwifruit
Lettuce
Mangos
Mushrooms

Onions
Parsnips
Pears
Peas
Potatoes
Pumpkins
Radishes
Raspberries

Rutabagas
Spinach
Sweet potatoes
Swiss chard
Turnips
Winter squash
Yams

Winter

Beets
Brussels sprouts
Cabbage
Collard greens
Grapefruit
Kale
Kiwifruit

Leeks
Onions
Oranges
Parsnips
Pears
Potatoes
Pumpkins

Rutabagas
Sweet potatoes
Swiss chard
Turnips
Winter squash

Year-Round

Apples
Avocados

Bananas
Carrots

Lemons
Limes

MIND DIET LIFESTYLE RECOMMENDATIONS

In addition to diet, there are important contributors to overall brain health, such as exercise, sleep, stress reduction, and social and intellectual stimulation. These are the components that paint a picture of your overall well-being and can reduce your risk of developing such chronic conditions as cardiovascular diseases, type 2 diabetes, obesity, and Alzheimer's disease. Perhaps you get enough sleep on a regular basis or have little trouble making social connections, and that's great! But if there is one area where you feel you could make an improvement, set a small goal to work on it. To help you keep track of your goals, I've included a Lifestyle Tracker Chart (page 214). This chart can be photocopied for you to use as an ongoing tool.

Exercise

One 2006 study published in the *Journals of Gerontology* suggests that aerobic fitness is associated with the preservation of brain tissue in aging men and women. Researchers concluded that aerobic fitness maintains and enhances central nervous system health and cognitive functioning in older adults. A review published in the *Mayo Clinic Proceedings* suggests that ongoing moderate-intensity physical exercise "should be considered a prescription for lowering cognitive risks and slowing cognitive decline across the age spectrum." Researchers believe that regular aerobic exercise, such as running, walking, biking, rowing, and swimming, can help protect brain function and cardiovascular health. There are no specific guidelines for frequency and duration of exercise to reduce the risk of cognitive decline, but the National Institutes of Health suggests that adults perform moderate-intensity aerobic exercise at least 2 hours and 30 minutes per week, or 30 minutes per day.

Hydration

We all know that adequate hydration is crucial for maintaining good health, as water is involved in nearly every function in the human body. Water protects body organs and tissues, helps the kidneys and liver flush out waste products, and helps dissolve nutrients so they're easily accessible to the body. For that reason, it is suggested that men consume 15½ cups of water per day and women consume 11½ cups of water per day. I suggest keeping a refillable water bottle with you and monitoring your urine color; colorless or light yellow urine means you're well-hydrated.

Sleep

A 2014 review published in *Nature* suggests that sleep deprivation increases the concentration of amyloid peptides in the brain that lead to the development of Alzheimer's disease, whereas getting adequate sleep has the opposite effect. As you age, it becomes more difficult to get a good night's sleep. Sleep apnea is a common condition in those who have chronic conditions like obesity and cardiovascular diseases, and it can deprive your body of oxygen and may have harmful effects on brain tissue. Therefore, if you have been diagnosed with sleep apnea, it's important to properly manage it, and if you haven't been diagnosed, it's important to reduce your risk of developing it by adopting healthy lifestyle habits. The National Institutes on Aging suggest that adults need seven to nine hours of sleep each night. They recommend setting a regular sleep schedule and routine; avoiding napping late in the afternoon, caffeine in the afternoon and evening, and large meals before bedtime; and keeping your room at a comfortable temperature to help you sleep well and let your brain rest and reset.

Stress Reduction and Mood

Both chronic stress and having a negative outlook on life can take a toll on your health. A 2003 study published in *Neurology* showed that those with high levels of psychological distress had twice the risk of developing Alzheimer's disease, in comparison to those with low levels of psychological distress. A 2012 study published in the *Archives of General Psychiatry* concluded that study participants who reported higher levels of purpose in life had better cognitive function and reduced risks of developing Alzheimer's

disease. Although it's easier said than done, reframing negative thoughts to positive ones can improve your overall health. In addition, stress-reduction activities such as exercising regularly; participating in relaxing activities such as yoga, meditation, or reading; and talking to a loved one can also improve your health. If stress and negative thoughts seem out of control and are impacting your daily life, I suggest seeking professional help.

Intellectually Stimulating Pursuits

Intellectually stimulating activities, such as playing word games, reading books, and learning to play an instrument, can impact cognition. Studies also show that having a robust social life and surrounding yourself with people you enjoy being around can also preserve cognitive function. Keep in mind, though, that studies also show that those with frequent negative social interactions have lower levels of cognition. The key here is to participate in a variety of mentally stimulating activities and maintain a positive social life.

It's important to consider your lifestyle habits over the long term versus the short term, meaning that, if you have one night of not-so-great sleep or one fast food meal over the course of several weeks, that's okay. How you take care of yourself over long periods of time and what you do most frequently will have the greatest impacts on your health.

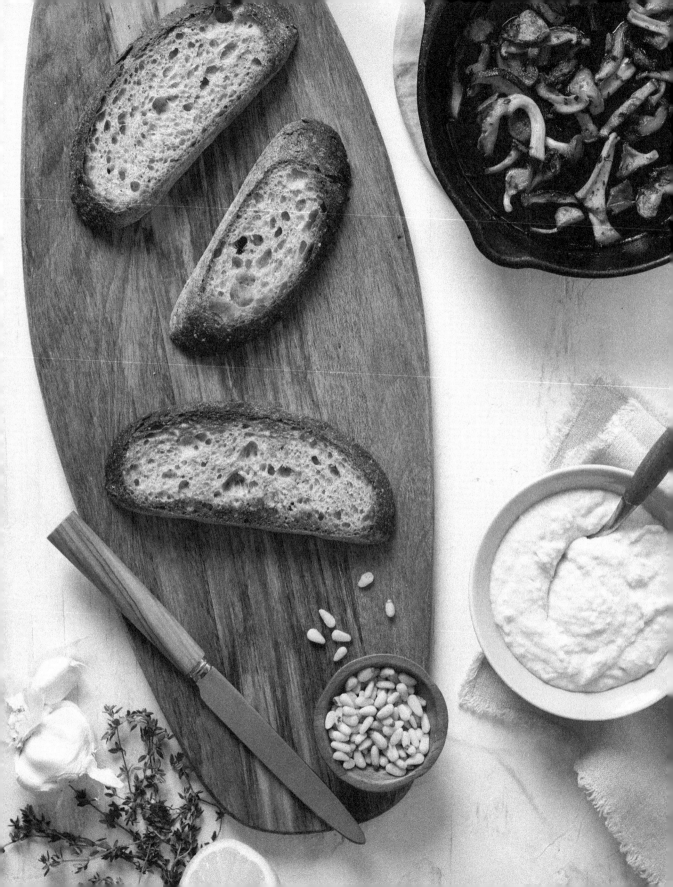

CHAPTER THREE

The MIND Diet Meal Plan

In this chapter, you'll learn how to put the MIND diet food recommendations into practice using a semi-structured meal plan. Meal plans are guides designed to help educate, inspire, and empower you to achieve your nutritional goals. They're meant to help you develop a routine that includes planning and prepping your meals and snacks. The one I designed for this book will also introduce you to new foods and recipes and show you how to incorporate the MIND diet superfoods into your everyday life. As you go through the meal plan, remember that it takes time to create new habits, and even if you don't follow it to the letter, you can still improve your overall health and reduce your risk of Alzheimer's disease and dementia by up to 53 percent! By the time you complete the following 28-day meal plan, I hope you feel confident crafting your own daily and weekly meal plans in a way that is sustainable in the long term for you and your family.

SETTING THE STAGE FOR YOUR MIND DIET

Food prep and cooking can seem daunting, especially if you consider yourself a novice in the kitchen. But with the simple and delicious MIND-friendly recipes and meal plan I've crafted for this book, I think you're going to find it easier to make healthy choices throughout the week. Here are some of my favorite aspects of meal planning:

It saves time. You often save time by spending a few hours each week prepping items like vegetables, fruits, grains, and meats. When these foods are readily available to make into meals and snacks, it's more convenient to make nutritious choices. I find it helpful to do the "heavy lifting," like chopping veggies and fruits, on the weekend when I have a bit more time, and then taking a few minutes on weekday evenings to assemble what I've prepped for dinner.

It saves money. Many people find that they save money by making a meal plan. Rather than shopping for random items at the grocery store that often go to waste, you purchase just the items you need for the week.

It helps achieve goals. When you make a meal plan and shopping list, you're more likely to achieve your goals, such as eating a cup of greens each day or eating fish once per week. If you don't have the right foods readily available, it's difficult to follow through with your goals.

It's flexible. Meal planning can be as strict or as flexible as you want it to be. Some people enjoy having a structured plan each week that they abide by, while others like to have healthy staples on hand and a loose idea of what they're going to cook, which can change day to day. There is no right or wrong way—it just depends on your style and what works for you and your family.

It reduces stress. "What's for dinner?" We've all been there, and it's not a great feeling. Uncertainty can contribute to unnecessary stress, so having at least a rough idea of what's for dinner before your week starts can lighten your load during the week. The scents, colors, and flavors of preparing mostly scratch-made meals can actually be a stress reliever, even if every meal doesn't turn out perfectly. It's the experience and

A NOTE ABOUT SODIUM

You may be wondering about sodium, since the MIND diet uses bits and pieces of the DASH diet, which is a lower-sodium diet designed to promote heart health. While the MIND diet doesn't provide specific recommendations for sodium intake, I suggest being mindful of how much salt you add to your food. As you'll see in my recipes, I almost always add salt because it enhances the flavor of food; without it, food tastes bland. Most of the foods I cook with and include in the MIND diet recipes are naturally low in sodium and high in nutrients that support heart health, such as potassium and fiber. Because our goal is to optimize heart health in order to preserve brain health, the recipes in this book all contain less than 30 percent of the daily recommended amount of sodium, as outlined in the Dietary Guidelines for Americans. You can decrease or increase the amount of salt you add to your food based on your personal needs and preferences. This is one of the many nutritional perks of cooking mostly from scratch—you're in charge!

BE PREPARED!

For each week of the Meal Plan, you'll find a shopping list and a handy prep list. These are meant to help you get organized and to save you time when making meals during the week. The prep lists include tasks tied to days of the week, but feel free to rearrange them to suit your schedule.

feeling of pride in cooking your own meals and snacks that will get your week started off on a positive note.

It adds variety. Meal planning gives you the opportunity to try new recipes and foods. Those who don't plan their meals in advance are more likely to eat the same things each week. And while there's nothing wrong with routine, it's good to introduce new, nutritious foods into your diet on a regular basis.

It's important to note that cooking more often doesn't mean you have to spend hours in front of the stove every night. But it does mean that you'll spend a little extra time prepping and cooking a few times each week to make life easier on other days. After a few weeks, it'll become routine and you'll figure out how to make modifications that best fit your lifestyle. Remember—it's not about perfection, just working to make better choices each and every day.

About the Recipes

It's time to get in the kitchen! The recipes in the following meal plan are all found in part two. They feature brain-healthy foods to help you achieve the daily and weekly nutritional goals outlined in the MIND diet; you'll find these ingredients highlighted in each recipe. In addition, you'll find Variation Tips to modify the recipes or change them up to keep things interesting. I also include Cooking Tips to help you gain skills and confidence in the kitchen. Finally, in several recipes, there are Make It a Meal Tips with pairing suggestions. Each recipe also includes helpful labels, so you can navigate whether a recipe is vegetarian or vegan, gluten-free, fast to prepare, or a one-pot meal. I hope you're as excited as I am to get cooking!

PANTRY, REFRIGERATOR, AND FREEZER STAPLES

Planning meals and snacks for the week becomes easier when you have a few staples in your pantry, fridge, and freezer. I've compiled a list of basic ingredients that you may want to have on hand; I did not include them in the weekly shopping lists that follow, since most of these items should always be stocked in your kitchen. Many of these items are building blocks for well-balanced meals, while other ingredients provide balance, add flavor, or give a boost of nutrition to your recipes. You certainly don't need all of these ingredients right away, but it's a good idea to build up your pantry over time so you have plenty of options.

Pantry:

OILS AND VINEGARS

Apple cider vinegar
Avocado oil or canola oil
Balsamic vinegar
Cooking spray
Extra-virgin olive oil
Red wine vinegar
Rice wine vinegar
Sesame oil
White wine vinegar

HERBS AND SPICES

Black pepper
Cayenne pepper
Chili powder
Crushed red pepper flakes
Dried dill
Dried oregano
Garam masala or
  ras el hanout
Garlic powder
Ground cinnamon
Ground cumin
Ground ginger
Ground nutmeg
Italian seasoning
Kosher salt or sea salt
Onion powder
Smoked paprika

NUTS, SEEDS, AND GRAINS

Assorted ancient grains
Assorted nuts and seeds
Brown rice
Chia seeds
Ground flaxseed
Old-fashioned rolled oats
Panko breadcrumbs
Quinoa
Sesame seeds

BAKING SUPPLIES

All-purpose flour
Baking powder
Baking soda
Cornstarch
Dark chocolate chips
Peanut butter or almond
  butter, natural
Pure vanilla extract
Raisins
Unsweetened
  shredded coconut
Whole wheat flour and/or
  whole wheat pastry flour
Yellow cornmeal

CANNED GOODS

Assorted canned beans

Crushed tomatoes

Diced tomatoes

Low-sodium bouillon

Tomato paste

Unsalted chicken stock and
   vegetable broth

SWEETENERS

Dark brown sugar

Granulated stevia

Granulated sugar

Honey

Refrigerator:

Dark leafy greens

Dijon mustard

Mayonnaise

Pure maple syrup

Salad greens

Sriracha sauce

Unsalted butter

Worcestershire sauce

Yellow mustard

Freezer:

Assorted fruit

Assorted vegetables

Berries

Dark leafy greens

Fish and seafood

Poultry, pork, and beef

Some of these foods, like berries, dark leafy greens, and meats, are also outlined in your meal plan. I've put them here in this section, as well, to reinforce that they should be staples in your daily and weekly meal plans.

WHAT IS STEVIA?

Stevia is an extract from the *Stevia rebaudiana* plant. It has become popular in recent years because it is a natural plant extract that is nonnutritive, meaning that it is calorie and sugar free. The FDA deems it Generally Recognized as Safe (GRAS), and it is manufactured and sold under many different brands, such as Truvia®, Pure Via®, SweetLeaf®, and Stevia in the Raw®. I use the granulated version in small amounts to sweeten smoothies, coffee, and tea. You can also use it in baking as a substitute for sugar, but note that it is 40 times sweeter than sugar, so use a conversion of 1 tablespoon granulated stevia for every ½ cup of sugar.

Week 1

"Simple ingredients prepared in a simple way—that's the best way to take your everyday cooking to a higher level."

—JOSÉ ANDRÉS, CHEF AND RESTAURATEUR

The first week of a meal plan is generally the most difficult, because it's a new regimen and a new set of nutrition recommendations. But what's also exciting about the first week is trying new foods and recipes, making a plan to set you up for success, and, my favorite— spending a little more time in the kitchen. You may go through this list, pick out a few things that you're really excited to try, and swap out others you may not be interested in. You may also decide that the recipes provided need to be doubled because you have a large family or cut in half because you're feeding only one or two people. Making modifications and developing your own personal plan is the ultimate goal of meal planning. The one I've provided here is simply to get you started, to give you some inspiration, and to guide you in eating in a more balanced way. It was specifically designed to fit the MIND diet foods into your daily and weekly meal routines. After all, your goal is to reduce your risk of Alzheimer's disease and dementia and to improve your overall health. I'm so excited to be on this journey with you, so let's get started!

Week 1 Shopping List

Produce:

- Avocados, 4
- Baby spinach, 12 to 13 cups
- Banana, 1
- Beet, 1
- Berries, assorted, 3 pints
- Cilantro, 1 bunch
- Dried Thai chiles, 2
- Fresh vegetables and fruit, as needed for snacks
- Garlic, 2 heads
- Ginger, 2-inch piece
- Green bell peppers, 2
- Green onions, 1 small bunch
- Kale, 1 large bunch
- Lemon, 1
- Limes, 2
- Mushrooms, 1 cup
- Oranges, 3
- Parsnips, 2
- Rainbow or Swiss chard, 1 large bunch
- Raspberries, 1 pint
- Red bell peppers, 2
- Red cabbage, shredded, ½ cup
- Red onions, 2
- Salsa, prepared, 1 small tub or jar
- Spring mix, 6 to 7 cups
- Sweet potatoes, 3
- Sweet Vidalia onion, 1
- Thyme, 1 small bunch
- Tofu, extra firm, 1 pound
- Yellow onions, 2

Dairy:

- Cheddar cheese, shredded, 2 tablespoons
- Eggs, large, 2 dozen
- Feta cheese, crumbled, ¼ cup
- Greek yogurt, plain, 4 cups
- Hummus, prepared, 1 small tub
- Milk of choice, 4½ cups
- Mozzarella, shredded, 2 cups
- Parmesan, freshly grated, ¼ cup

Meat, Poultry, and Fish:

- Chicken breast, boneless, skinless, 1 pound
- Pork shoulder, 1½ pounds
- Salmon fillets, 1 pound
- Turkey breakfast sausage links, 1 (12-ounce) package
- Turkey sausage, 2 pounds

Canned/Dried Goods:

- Black or green olives, sliced, ½ cup
- Marinara, low sodium, 1 (24-ounce) jar
- No-salt-added black beans, 3 (15-ounce) cans
- No-salt-added dark red kidney beans, 1 (15-ounce) can
- No-salt-added fire-roasted diced tomatoes, 2 (15-ounce) cans
- No-salt-added pinto beans, 1 (15-ounce) can
- Roasted red peppers, 1 small jar
- Whole-grain orzo, ¾ cup
- Whole-grain ziti or other shaped pasta, 12 ounces

Frozen:

- Cauliflower florets, 2 cups
- Dark sweet cherries, 3 cups
- Hash browns or cubed potatoes, 2 cups

Other:

- Corn tortillas, 16 (6-inch)
- Dark chocolate chips, 1 small bag
- Mixed nuts, as needed for snacks
- Peanuts, ½ cup
- Tortilla chips, 1 (12-ounce) bag
- Unsalted broth of choice, 2 (32-ounce) containers
- Walnuts or pecans, ¼ cup
- Whole-grain baguette, 2

Week 1
Meal Plan

	Monday	*Tuesday*	*Wednesday*
BREAKFAST	• Mini Spinach and Potato Frittatas (page 72) • 1 medium piece of fruit or ½ cup berries	• Cherry-Oat Smoothie (page 66)	• Leftover Mini Spinach and Potato Frittatas (page 72) • 1 medium piece of fruit or ½ cup berries
LUNCH	• Triple Berry Chicken Salad (page 80)	• Leftover Honey Mustard Grilled Salmon (page 152) • Leftover Roasted Balsamic Root Vegetables (page 98) • 1 to 2 cups spring mix • 2 tablespoons vinaigrette dressing (see "For the dressing" on page 82)	• Leftover Three-Bean and Vegetable Chili (page 90) • Whole-grain baguette (3- to 4-inch piece)
DINNER	• Honey Mustard Grilled Salmon (page 152) • Roasted Balsamic Root Vegetables (page 98) • ½ to 1 cup sautéed leafy green vegetables with garlic	• Three-Bean and Vegetable Chili (page 90) • Whole-grain baguette, (3- to 4-inch piece)	• Crispy Pork and Avocado Tacos (page 184) • 1 cup roasted, sautéed, or grilled vegetables
DESSERT			
SNACKS (2-3 throughout the day)	• 1 ounce nuts plus 1 cup fruit or ½ cup berries • 2 tablespoons nut butter plus 1 banana or apple • ¼ cup hummus plus 1 cup veggies	• See Monday's snack list	• See Monday's snack list

Week 1 Prep List

SUNDAY:

• prep the fruits and vegetables for meals and side dishes for the week by chopping them and placing them in containers or zip-top plastic bags.

• prep snacks by placing nuts in sealed plastic bags and nut butter and hummus in small containers, and chopping fruits and vegetables and placing them in small containers or sealed plastic bags.

• make the Mini Spinach and Potato Frittatas, place them in microwave-safe containers, and refrigerate.

Thursday	Friday	Saturday	Sunday
• Cherry-Oat Smoothie (page 66)	• Leftover Mini Spinach and Potato Frittatas (page 72) • 1 medium piece of fruit or ½ cup berries	• Raspberry-Honey Pancakes (page 68) • 2 links turkey or veggie break-fast sausage	• Rainbow Chard and Sweet Potato Hash (page 74) • 1 medium piece of fruit or ½ cup berries
• Leftover Crispy Pork and Avocado Tacos (page 184) • 1 cup roasted, sautéed, or grilled vegetables	• Leftover Kung Pao Tofu Stir-Fry (page 120) • 1 cup sautéed leafy green vegetables with garlic	• Leftover Turkey Sausage and Kale Baked Ziti (page 178) • 1 cup roasted, sautéed, or grilled vegetables	• Italian Wedding Soup (page 94) • Whole-grain baguette (3- to 4-inch piece)
• Kung Pao Tofu Stir-Fry (page 120) • ½ to 1 cup sautéed leafy green vegetables with garlic	• Turkey Sausage and Kale Baked Ziti (page 178) • 1 cup roasted, sautéed, or grilled vegetables	• Black Bean Nachos (page 108) • 1 to 2 cups spring mix • 2 tablespoons vinaigrette dressing (see "For the dressing" on page 82)	• Veggie Pizza with Creamy Cauliflower Sauce (page 128) • 1 to 2 cups spring mix • 2 tablespoons vinaigrette dressing (see "For the dressing" on page 82)
		• Chocolate Avocado Mousse (page 206)	• Leftover Chocolate Avocado Mousse (page 206)
• See Monday's snack list	• See Monday's snack list	• See Monday's snack list	• See Monday's snack list

• cook the chicken for the Triple Berry Chicken Salad, place it in an airtight container, and refrigerate.

• chop the vegetables for the Roasted Balsamic Root Vegetables, place them in containers, and refrigerate.

WEDNESDAY:

• in the morning, prep the pork for the Crispy Pork and Avocado Tacos and cook it in the slow cooker (follow the Cooking Tip directions for the slow cooker method).

• at night, prep the stir-fry sauce and cook the rice for Kung Pao Tofu Stir-Fry.

• take inventory of your prepped vegetables, fruits, and snacks, and prep any additional.

Week 2

"One of the most meditative times of my day is when I'm cooking."

—GABRIELLE BERNSTEIN, MOTIVATIONAL SPEAKER AND AUTHOR

If you're like me and most other people, you'll likely note that your first week following this MIND diet meal plan was not perfect. That's absolutely okay, and a normal part of life! The goal is not for you to achieve perfection now or later. I'm just looking to help you cook more, eat more MIND diet superfoods, and make small, lasting changes that can help improve your brain health. If you ate a cup or two of berries, a handful of greens, or swapped out white bread for whole grain, you're well on your way! These types of changes are the ones that will make a great impact on your health over time. Let's head into week 2 and try some new recipes!

Week 2 Shopping List

Produce:

- Apples, 4
- Avocados, 2
- Baby spinach, 5 to 6 cups
- Basil, 1 small bunch
- Berries, assorted, 2 to 3 pints
- Bibb lettuce, 2 to 3 heads
- Blueberries, 4 cups
- Cabbage, 1 head or 1 (10-ounce) bag coleslaw mix
- Carrots, 2
- Cauliflower florets, 4 to 5 cups
- Celery, 1 small bunch
- Cilantro, 2 bunches
- English cucumber, 1
- Fresh vegetables and fruit, as needed for snacks
- Garlic, 1 head
- Ginger, 3-inch piece
- Green onions, 1 small bunch
- Italian parsley, 1 bunch
- Jalapeños, 2
- Kale, 1 large bunch
- Lemons, 3
- Limes, 4
- Mint, 1 small bunch
- Oranges, 6
- Oregano, 1 small bunch
- Red bell pepper, 1
- Rosemary, 1 small bunch
- Spring mix, 4 to 5 cups
- Sweet potatoes, 6
- Yellow onions, 4
- Zucchini, 1

Dairy:

- Eggs, large, 15
- Greek yogurt, plain, 1 cup
- Greek yogurt, vanilla or fruit-flavored, 7 to 8 cups
- Heavy cream or half-and-half, 3 tablespoons
- Milk of choice, ½ cup
- Parmesan, freshly grated, 1 cup
- Yogurt (not Greek-style), plain, 2 tablespoons

Meat, Poultry, and Fish:

- Ground turkey, 1½ pounds
- Lean ground beef, 1 pound
- Pork tenderloin, 2 pounds
- White fish, 1½ pounds

Canned/Dried Goods:

- Corn tortillas, 12 (6-inch)
- Crushed pineapple, 1 small can
- Crushed tomatoes, 1 (28-ounce) can
- No-salt-added cannellini beans, 2 (15-ounce) cans
- No-salt-added chickpeas, 1 (15-ounce) can
- Salmon, canned or pouched, 20 ounces

Frozen:

- Berries, assorted, 2 cups
- Cauliflower florets, 4 to 5 cups
- Dark sweet cherries, 3 cups
- Hash browns or cubed potatoes, 2 cups
- Mixed vegetables, 4 cups

Other:

- Fish sauce, 1 small bottle
- Nuts, assorted (almonds, pecans, walnuts), 2¼ cups
- Unsalted chicken stock or vegetable broth, 2 (32-ounce) containers
- Walnuts, chopped, 2½ cups
- Whole-grain bread, 1 loaf
- Whole-grain pitas, 1 pack

Week 2
Meal Plan

	Monday	*Tuesday*	*Wednesday*
BREAKFAST	• Leftover Rainbow Chard and Sweet Potato Hash (page 74) • 1 medium piece of fruit or ½ cup berries	• Blueberry, Orange, and Granola Parfait (page 64)	• Blueberry, Orange, and Granola Parfait (page 64)
LUNCH	• Leftover Italian Wedding Soup (page 94) • Whole-grain baguette (3- to 4-inch piece)	• Leftover Thai-Style Cauliflower-Walnut Lettuce Cups (page 134)	• Leftover Fish Tacos with Cabbage Slaw (page 160) • 1 medium piece of fruit or ½ cup berries
DINNER	• Thai-Style Cauliflower-Walnut Lettuce Cups (page 134)	• Fish Tacos with Cabbage Slaw (page 160) • 1 medium piece of fruit or ½ cup berries	• Turkey-Zucchini Meat Loaf (page 176) • Tomato-Basil Bisque (page 92) • 1 to 2 cups spring mix • 2 tablespoons vinaigrette dressing (see "For the dressing" on page 82)
DESSERT			
SNACKS (2-3 throughout the day)	• ½ cup yogurt plus ½ cup berries • Salmon Salad Sandwiches (page 156) • Carrot Cake-Walnut Muffins (page 210)	• See Monday's snack list	• See Monday's snack list

Week 2 Prep List

SUNDAY:

• prep the fruits and vegetables for meals and side dishes for the week by chopping them and placing them in containers or zip-top plastic bags. Also, prep snacks by placing the berries in containers.

• prep the salad for Salmon Salad Sandwiches and make the Carrot Cake-Walnut Muffins.

• make the granola for Blueberry, Orange, and Granola Parfait.

	Thursday	Friday	Saturday	Sunday
	• Peanut Butter–Berry Overnight Oats (page 67)	• Peanut Butter–Berry Overnight Oats (page 67)	• Shakshuka with Poached Eggs (page 76) • 1 medium piece of fruit or ½ cup berries	• 2 egg scramble with 1 cup veggies • 1 slice whole-grain toast with 1 teaspoon unsalted butter
	• Leftover Turkey Zucchini Meat Loaf (page 176) • Leftover Tomato-Basil Bisque (page 92) • 1 to 2 cups spring mix • 2 tablespoons vinaigrette dressing (see "For the dressing" on page 82)	• Leftover Garlicky White Bean Cassoulet (page 114) • 1 medium piece of fruit or ½ cup berries	• Leftover Cuban-Style Mojo Pork Tenderloin (page 188) • 1 medium cooked sweet potato with 1 teaspoon unsalted butter and ground cinnamon • ½ to 1 cup sautéed leafy green vegetables with garlic	• Leftover Baked Chickpea and Spinach Falafel (page 110) • 1 whole-grain pita • ¼ cup sliced cucumbers • 2 tablespoons plain Greek yogurt
	• Garlicky White Bean Cassoulet (page 114) • 1 medium piece of fruit or ½ cup berries	• Cuban-Style Mojo Pork Tenderloin (page 188) • 1 medium cooked sweet potato with 1 teaspoon unsalted butter and ground cinnamon • ½ to 1 cup sautéed leafy green vegetables with garlic	• Baked Chickpea and Spinach Falafel (page 110) • 1 whole-grain pita • ¼ cup sliced cucumbers • 2 tablespoons plain Greek yogurt	• Beef and Sweet Potato Shepherd's Pie (page 190) • 1 to 2 cups spring mix • 2 tablespoons vinaigrette dressing (see "For the dressing" on page 82)
			• Crustless Apple Pies (page 212)	• Crustless Apple Pies (page 212)
	• See Monday's snack list	• See Monday's snack list	• See Monday's snack list	• See Monday's snack list

TUESDAY (NIGHT):

• prep for the Turkey Zucchini Meat Loaf by shredding the zucchini and mixing together the ingredients for the Meat Loaf; refrigerate the meat mixture, then bake it on Wednesday night.

• make the Tomato-Basil Bisque; refrigerate it, then reheat it on Wednesday night.

WEDNESDAY (NIGHT):

• make the Peanut Butter–Berry Overnight Oats.

Week 3

"When you have good ingredients, cooking doesn't require a lot of instruction because you can never go wrong."

—ALICE WATERS, CHEF, AUTHOR, AND FOOD ACTIVIST

As you work through the meal plans to figure out what works best, you may find that you have some leftover meals and ingredients in your fridge; now is the time to plan those into next week's meals and snacks. If you have a leftover pepper, half a container of spinach, and some eggs, that's totally normal. Add the bell pepper to your Rainbow Veggie Spring Rolls (page 132), blend some spinach into your smoothie, and hard-boil the eggs for on-the-go snacks. You can also pop most leftovers into the freezer to eat at a later time. With a little planning, there are ways to reduce waste and incorporate more veggies and other nutritious foods into next week's plan. You may also be wondering how to fit restaurant meals or party foods into a balanced plan. My best advice is to enjoy your favorite foods in moderation, and move on to your normal routine afterward. Dining out and enjoying party foods are normal parts of life, and they're meant to be enjoyed without extra stress. Onward!

Week 3 Shopping List

Produce:

- Avocados, 6
- Baby spinach, 12 to 13 cups
- Bananas, 2
- Berries, assorted, 2 to 3 pints
- Butternut squash, 1
- Carrots, 3
- Cilantro, 1 bunch
- Dill, 1 small bunch
- English cucumber, 2
- Fennel, 1 bulb
- Fresh vegetables and fruit, as needed for snacks
- Garlic, 1 head
- Ginger, 6-inch piece
- Green onions, 1 bunch
- Italian parsley, 2 bunches
- Jalapeño, 1
- Lemons, 7
- Limes, 6
- Oranges, 3
- Red bell pepper, 1
- Roma tomatoes, 4
- Shallots, 2
- Shredded purple cabbage, 1 cup
- Spring mix, 4 to 5 cups
- Strawberries, 2 pints
- Sugar snap peas, ½ cup
- Yellow onions, 3
- Zucchini, 2

Dairy:

- Eggs, large, 1 dozen
- Greek yogurt, plain, 3 cups
- Greek yogurt, vanilla, ½ cup
- Low-fat cream cheese, 8 ounces
- Milk of choice, 5 cups
- Yogurt (not Greek-style), plain, 2 tablespoons

Meat, Poultry, and Fish:

- Ahi tuna, 1 pound
- Chicken breasts, boneless, skinless, 2 pounds
- Chicken thighs, boneless, skinless, 2 pounds
- Raw shrimp, 16–20 count, peeled and deveined, 3 pounds
- Scallops, large, 1 pound
- Turkey or veggie breakfast sausage links, 1 (12-ounce) package

Canned/Dried Goods:

- Brown rice noodles, 8 ounces
- Bulgur, 1 cup
- Farro, 2 cups
- Full-fat coconut milk, 1 (15-ounce) can
- No-salt-added chickpeas, 2 (15-ounce) cans
- Pumpkin purée, 1 (15-ounce) can
- Red or green lentils, 1 cup

Frozen:

- Dark sweet cherries, 3 cups
- Hash browns or cubed potatoes, 2 cups

Other:

- Graham crackers, 1 small box
- Orange preserves, 1 small jar
- Peanuts, ½ cup
- Pistachios, ½ cup
- Poppy seeds, 1 small container
- Sliced unsalted almonds, ½ cup
- Spring roll wrappers/rice paper, 1 package
- Sweet chili sauce, 1 small jar
- Unsalted chicken stock or vegetable broth, 2 (32-ounce) containers
- Walnuts, chopped, ½ cup
- Whole pitted green olives, ½ cup
- Whole-grain bread, 1 loaf

Week 3
Meal Plan

	Monday	*Tuesday*	*Wednesday*
BREAKFAST	• Cherry-Oat Smoothie (page 66)	• Mini Spinach and Potato Frittatas (page 72) • 1 medium piece of fruit or ½ cup berries	• Cherry-Oat Smoothie (page 66)
LUNCH	• Leftover Beef and Sweet Potato Shepherd's Pie (page 190) • ½ to 1 cup sautéed leafy green vegetables with garlic	• Leftover Tuna Burgers with Scallion Aioli (page 148) • 1 to 2 cups spring mix • 2 tablespoons vinaigrette dressing (see "For the dressing" on page 82)	• Leftover Greek-Style Lemon Chicken and Rice Skillet (page 168) • 1 cup roasted, sautéed, or grilled vegetables
DINNER	• Tuna Burgers with Scallion Aioli (page 148) • 1 to 2 cups spring mix • 2 tablespoons vinaigrette dressing (see "For the dressing" on page 82)	• Greek-Style Lemon Chicken and Rice Skillet (page 168) • 1 cup roasted, sautéed, or grilled vegetables	• Citrus-Marinated Coconut Shrimp (page 146) • Spinach, Strawberry, and Fennel Salad (page 85)
DESSERT			
SNACKS (2-3 throughout the day)	• 1 slice whole-grain toast plus ⅓ mashed avocado • 2 Rainbow Veggie Spring Rolls (page 132) • Pumpkin Oatmeal Raisin Cookies (page 204)	• See Monday's snack list	• See Monday's snack list

Week 3 Prep List

SUNDAY:
- prep the fruit and vegetables for meals and side dishes for the week by chopping them and placing them in containers or zip-top plastic bags.
- prep snacks by making the Rainbow Veggie Spring Rolls and Pumpkin Oatmeal Raisin Cookies.
- make the Mini Spinach and Potato Frittatas, place them in microwave-safe containers, and refrigerate.

TUESDAY (NIGHT):
- marinate the Citrus-Marinated Coconut Shrimp; refrigerate, then finish cooking the recipe on Wednesday night.

Thursday	Friday	Saturday	Sunday
• Leftover Mini Spinach and Potato Frittatas (page 72) • 1 medium piece of fruit or ½ cup berries	• Cherry-Oat Smoothie (page 66)	• Banana-Nut Breakfast Porridge (page 70) • 2 links turkey or veggie breakfast sausage	• 2 egg omelet with ½ to 1 cup sautéed leafy green vegetables • 1 slice whole-grain toast with 1 teaspoon unsalted butter
• Leftover Citrus-Marinated Coconut Shrimp (page 146) • Leftover Spinach, Strawberry and Fennel Salad (page 85)	• Leftover Moroccan-Style Chicken Tagine (page 170) • 1 medium piece of fruit or ½ cup berries	• Leftover Zucchini-Lentil Fritters (page 118) • Leftover Classic Tabbouleh (page 84)	• Leftover Shrimp-Peanut Pad Thai (page 142) • 1 medium piece of fruit or ½ cup berries
• Moroccan-Style Chicken Tagine (page 170) • 1 medium piece of fruit or ½ cup berries	• Zucchini-Lentil Fritters (page 118) • Classic Tabbouleh (page 84)	• Shrimp-Peanut Pad Thai (page 142) • 1 medium piece of fruit or ½ cup berries	• Pistachio-Crusted Scallops (page 164) • Maple Butternut Squash Soup (page 96)
		• Mini Strawberry Cheesecake Parfaits (page 207)	• Mini Strawberry Cheesecake Parfaits (page 207)
• See Monday's snack list	• See Monday's snack list	• See Monday's snack list	• See Monday's snack list

WEDNESDAY (NIGHT):
• marinate the Moroccan-Style Chicken Tagine; refrigerate, then finish cooking the recipe on Thursday night.

THURSDAY (NIGHT):
• cook the bulgur for the Classic Tabbouleh, and refrigerate.
• cook the lentils for the Zucchini-Lentil Fritters, and refrigerate.

Week 4

"You don't have to cook fancy or complicated masterpieces—just good food with fresh ingredients."

—JULIA CHILD, CHEF, AUTHOR, TV PERSONALITY

It's week 4, and you're a culinary rockstar! At this point, I hope you feel you have improved your skills in the kitchen and have some new, delicious recipes to keep in your back pocket. Going forward, your meal plan may not look exactly like the plan I've outlined, but I encourage you to focus on continuing to include the MIND diet foods in your rotation, to cook your own meals most of the time, and to try new recipes on a regular basis. Remember that eating in a nutritious and balanced way doesn't have to be complicated or unpleasant. I hope the recipes you've tried and your journey so far have left you feeling nourished, inspired, satisfied, and excited for what's to come.

Week 4 Shopping List

Produce:
- Asparagus, 1 pound
- Avocados, 2
- Baby spinach, 7 to 8 cups
- Bartlett pear, 1
- Berries, assorted, 1 to 2 pints
- Broccoli, 1 head
- Butternut squash, 2
- Cilantro, 2 bunches
- Garlic, 1 head
- Ginger, 5-inch piece
- Green bell pepper, 1
- Green onions, 1 bunch
- Italian parsley, 1 bunch
- Jalapeño, 1
- Kale, 1 bunch
- Lemons, 5
- Limes, 1
- Mushrooms, 2 cups
- Oranges, 3
- Rainbow or Swiss chard, 1 bunch
- Red bell peppers, 2
- Red onion, 1
- Spring mix, 4 to 5 cups
- Sweet potato, 1
- Sweet Vidalia onion, 1
- Thyme, 1 small bunch
- Yellow onions, 3

Dairy:
- Eggs, large, 32
- Greek yogurt, plain, ½ cup
- Mexican-style cheese blend, shredded, 1 cup
- Milk of choice, 3½ cups
- Parmesan, freshly grated, ½ cup

Meat, Poultry, and Fish:
- Chicken breast, boneless, skinless, 1½ pounds
- Lean ground beef, 1 pound
- Salmon fillets, 1½ pounds
- White fish, 1½ pounds
- Turkey or veggie breakfast sausage links, 1 (12-ounce) package

Canned/Dried Goods:
- Anchovy paste, 1 small tube
- Dill pickle relish, 1 small jar
- Enchilada sauce, ½ cup
- Farro, 2 cups
- Full-fat coconut milk, 1 (15-ounce) can
- Lump crab, canned, 12 ounces
- No-salt-added chickpeas, 3 (15-ounce) cans
- No-salt-added crushed tomatoes, 1 (28-ounce) can
- No-salt-added petite diced tomatoes, 1 (15-ounce) can
- Tortilla chips, 1 large bag
- Tuna, canned or pouched, 12 ounces
- Turbinado sugar, ½ tablespoon
- Unsweetened applesauce, 1 cup

Frozen:
- Mixed berries or blackberries, 2½ cups

Other:
- Dry white wine, 1 bottle
- Peanuts or cashews, ½ cup
- Sliced unsalted almonds, ¾ cup
- Unsalted chicken stock or vegetable broth, 3 (32-ounce) containers
- Walnuts, chopped, ½ cup
- Whole-grain baguette, 1
- Whole-grain crackers, 1 box

Week 4
Meal Plan

	Monday	*Tuesday*	*Wednesday*
BREAKFAST	• Peanut Butter–Berry Overnight Oats (page 67) • 2 links turkey or veggie breakfast sausage	• Peanut Butter–Berry Overnight Oats (page 67) • 2 links turkey or veggie breakfast sausage	• Peanut Butter–Berry Overnight Oats (page 67) • 2 links turkey or veggie breakfast sausage
LUNCH	• Leftover Maple Butternut Squash Soup (page 96) • Whole-grain baguette (3- to 4-inch piece)	• Leftover Vietnamese-Style Pork Meatball Bowls (page 186)	• Leftover Chickpea Coconut Curry (page 112) • 1 to 2 cups spring mix • 2 tablespoons vinaigrette dressing (see "For the dressing" on page 82)
DINNER	• Vietnamese-Style Pork Meatball Bowls (page 186)	• Chickpea Coconut Curry (page 112) • 1 to 2 cups spring mix • 2 tablespoons vinaigrette dressing (see "For the dressing" on page 82)	• Sesame-Ginger Glazed Salmon (page 154) • Asparagus Farro Risotto (page 126) • ½ to 1 cup sautéed leafy green vegetables with garlic
DESSERT			
SNACKS (2-3 throughout the day)	• 2 tablespoons nut butter plus 8 whole-grain crackers • Tuna and Avocado Egg Salad (page 150) • Cinnamon-Pear Snack Cake (page 208)	• See Monday's snack list	• See Monday's snack list

Week 4 Prep List

SUNDAY:

• prep the fruit and vegetables for the meals and side dishes for the week by chopping them and placing them in containers or zip-top plastic bags. Also prep the snacks by placing nut butter and crackers in containers.

• make the Tuna and Avocado Egg Salad and the Cinnamon-Pear Snack Cake.

• make the Peanut Butter–Berry Overnight Oats, and refrigerate.

• make the meatballs and rice, and prep the pickled veggies for Vietnamese-Style Pork Meatball Bowls.

Thursday	Friday	Saturday	Sunday
• Rainbow Chard and Sweet Potato Hash (page 74) • 1 medium piece of fruit or ½ cup berries	• Leftover Rainbow Chard and Sweet Potato Hash (page 74) • 1 medium piece fruit or ½ cup berries	• Egg scramble with 1 cup vegetables • 1 slice whole-grain toast with 1 teaspoon unsalted butter	• Shakshuka with Poached Eggs (page 76) • 1 medium piece of fruit or ½ cup berries
• Leftover Sesame-Ginger Glazed Salmon (page 154) • Leftover Asparagus Farro Risotto (page 126) • ½ to 1 cup sautéed leafy green vegeta	• Leftover Beef and Rice Fajita Casserole (page 194) • 8 tortilla chips	• Leftover White Fish Nuggets (page 158) • Leftover Kale and Crispy Chickpea Caesar Salad (page 86)	• Leftover Almond-Crusted Crab Cakes (page 157) • Leftover Cinnamon-Roasted Butternut Squash (page 100) • 1 cup roasted, sautéed, or grilled vegetables
• Beef and Rice Fajita Casserole (page 194) • 8 tortilla chips	• White Fish Nuggets (page 158) • Kale and Crispy Chickpea Caesar Salad (page 86)	• Almond-Crusted Crab Cakes (page 157) • Cinnamon-Roasted Butternut Squash (page 100) • 1 cup roasted, sautéed, or grilled vegetables	• Orange Chicken and Broccoli Stir-Fry (page 172)
		• Blackberry-Lemon Galette (page 202)	• Blackberry-Lemon Galette (page 202)
• See Monday's snack list	• See Monday's snack list	• See Monday's snack list	• See Monday's snack list

WEDNESDAY (NIGHT):
• make the Rainbow Chard and Sweet Potato Hash, and refrigerate.
• make the rice for Beef and Rice Fajita Casserole, and refrigerate.

Meal Plan

	Monday	*Tuesday*	*Wednesday*	
BREAKFAST				
LUNCH				
DINNER				
DESSERT				
SNACKS (2-3 throughout the day)				

BEYOND THE 28 DAYS

As I've mentioned many times, this meal plan is meant solely as a resource and guide to help you put the MIND diet recommendations into practice. As you made your way through the 28 days, you likely made some adjustments to fit your lifestyle, which is exactly what I was hoping you'd do. It's important to continue to plan what you're going to eat for the week—whether in a structured or more flexible way—and to continue to build a healthy pantry, refrigerator, and freezer.

Keep in mind that the MIND diet is an inclusive eating plan that encourages a wide variety of foods and is among the easiest to follow long-term. The goal is to consume plenty of vegetables and dark leafy greens, berries, whole grains, beans

	Thursday	Friday	Saturday	Sunday

and legumes, fish and seafood, poultry, and vegetable oils, while enjoying foods like red meat, butter, cheese, and sweets on occasion. There are plenty of ways to accomplish this, and it will be a continuous journey to achieve your goals.

For use as an ongoing tool, I have included a blank template for you to create your own custom meal plan. In part two, you'll find additional delicious MIND diet-friendly recipes that are not included in the meal plan in this chapter, but that you can easily plug in when you draw up your own personalized plan. You can photocopy the blank meal plan or download it from CallistoMediaBooks.com/MINDDiet. Cheers to better health and delicious food!

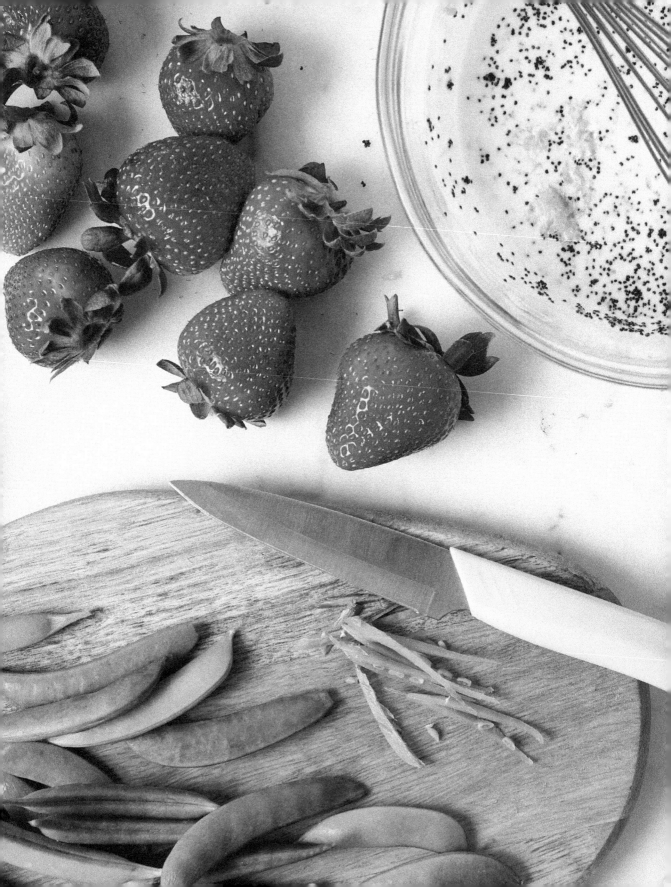

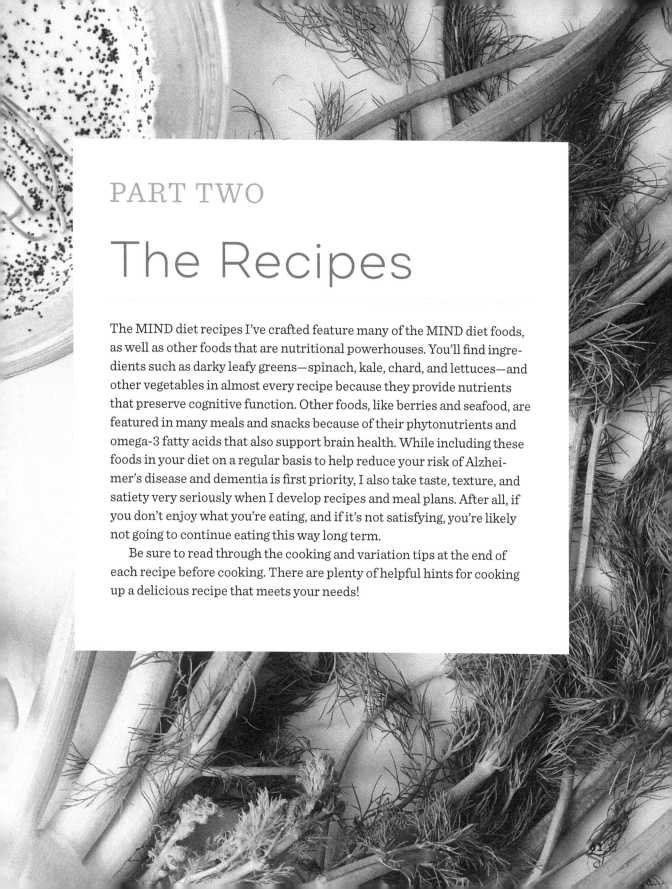

PART TWO

The Recipes

The MIND diet recipes I've crafted feature many of the MIND diet foods, as well as other foods that are nutritional powerhouses. You'll find ingredients such as darky leafy greens—spinach, kale, chard, and lettuces—and other vegetables in almost every recipe because they provide nutrients that preserve cognitive function. Other foods, like berries and seafood, are featured in many meals and snacks because of their phytonutrients and omega-3 fatty acids that also support brain health. While including these foods in your diet on a regular basis to help reduce your risk of Alzheimer's disease and dementia is first priority, I also take taste, texture, and satiety very seriously when I develop recipes and meal plans. After all, if you don't enjoy what you're eating, and if it's not satisfying, you're likely not going to continue eating this way long term.

Be sure to read through the cooking and variation tips at the end of each recipe before cooking. There are plenty of helpful hints for cooking up a delicious recipe that meets your needs!

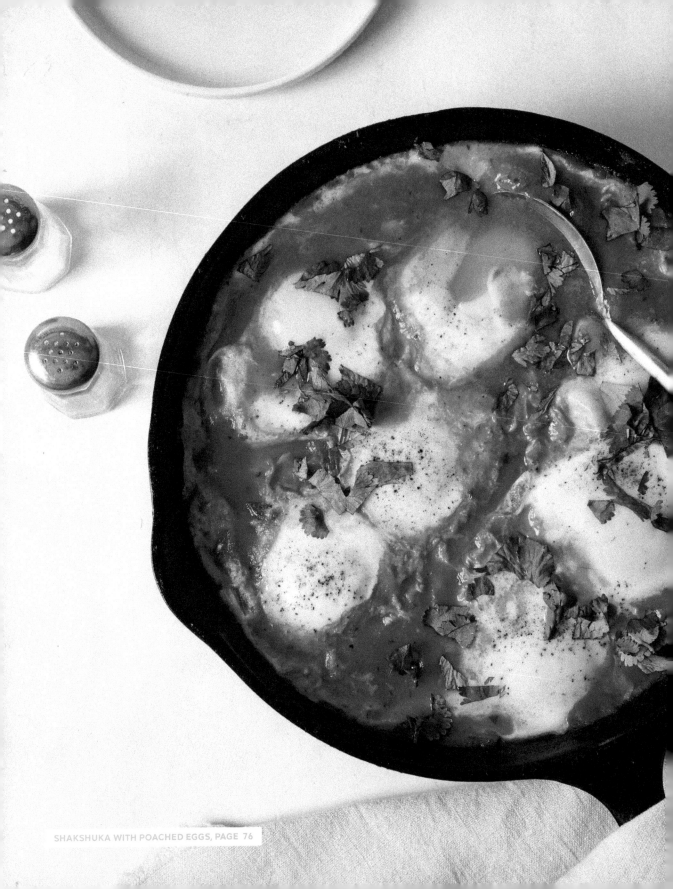

CHAPTER FOUR

Breakfast

BLUEBERRY, ORANGE, AND GRANOLA PARFAIT

SERVES 4 / PREP TIME: 10 MINUTES / COOK TIME: 1 HOUR

Making your own granola is simple and requires just a few ingredients, most of which are probably already in your pantry. It can be made in advance, and layered with yogurt and fruit to make a tasty parfait like this one, providing fiber and healthy fats to round out a balanced meal. Try any combination of fruits; the variations are endless.

For the granola

2 tablespoons honey or pure maple syrup

2 tablespoons avocado oil or canola oil

¼ teaspoon ground cinnamon

⅛ teaspoon kosher salt

2 cups old-fashioned rolled oats

½ cup chopped unsalted nuts

For the parfait

2 cups plain or vanilla Greek yogurt

2 cups blueberries

2 medium oranges, peeled and segmented

To make the granola

1. Preheat the oven to 250°F. Line a baking sheet with parchment paper; set aside.

2. In a medium bowl, whisk together the honey or maple syrup, oil, cinnamon, and salt. Stir in the oats and nuts until combined. Spread the granola mixture on the parchment paper and press it down into one solid layer.

3. Bake for 1 hour, stirring every 15 minutes, until the granola is lightly toasted. Remove it from the oven and let it cool completely, then break it into clusters.

To make the parfait

1. Spoon ¼ cup of yogurt into each of four tall glasses. Scoop ¼ cup blueberries, ¼ of the orange segments, and ¼ cup granola on top of each serving, then repeat the layers of yogurt, blueberries, oranges, and granola one more time.

2. The granola can be prepped in advance and stored at room temperature in a large sealed plastic bag or airtight container for up to two weeks. Assemble the parfaits just before eating to avoid the granola becoming soggy.

Variation Tip: Swap out the cow's milk yogurt for almond, coconut, or soy milk yogurt. Try raspberries or strawberries instead of blueberries.

Cooking Tip: To segment an orange, use a paring knife to slice the top and bottom off the orange. Slice the peel away from the flesh. Cut between the white membranes to segment the orange. Discard the membranes.

Nutrition Information (per serving): Calories 334; Total fat 13g; Saturated fat 2g; Cholesterol 5mg; Sodium 86mg; Carbs 44g; Fiber 6g; Sugar 22g; Protein 14g

CHERRY-OAT SMOOTHIES

SERVES 2 / PREP TIME: 10 MINUTES

Smoothies are a quick and easy way to pack nutrition into meals or snacks. If you're not usually a fan of dark leafy green vegetables, adding them to a smoothie with fruit typically masks the flavor. The oats boost the fiber content and add bulk, helping you stay full and satisfied for hours.

1½ cups milk

½ cup nonfat vanilla or plain Greek yogurt

1 medium banana, peeled and frozen

1½ cups frozen dark sweet cherries

1 cup baby spinach or chopped kale leaves

½ cup old-fashioned rolled oats

1 teaspoon granulated stevia

1. Place the milk, yogurt, banana, cherries, spinach or kale, oats, and stevia in the pitcher of a blender. Purée until smooth.

2. Serve immediately.

Variation Tip: Swap out the cow's milk yogurt for almond, coconut, or soy milk yogurt. Add 1 to 2 scoops of protein powder for an extra boost of lasting energy. Or add 1 to 2 tablespoons of ground flaxseed for a boost of fiber and omega-3s.

Cooking Tip: Peel and slice the bananas, place them in small sealable plastic bags, and store them in the freezer for easy smoothie prep.

Nutrition Information (per serving): Calories 246; Total fat 2g; Saturated fat 0g; Cholesterol 7mg; Sodium 109mg; Carbs 43g; Fiber 5g; Sugar 25g; Protein 16g

PEANUT BUTTER–BERRY OVERNIGHT OATS

SERVES 6 / PREP TIME: 10 MINUTES / CHILLING TIME: 4 HOURS

With this recipe, I've transformed the classic PB&J into a delicious bowl of overnight oatmeal. If you've never made them, overnight oats are as simple as whisking ingredients in a bowl, placing them in jars, and refrigerating them overnight. Scoop on some toppings—voilà!—breakfast is served.

3 cups milk

2 cups old-fashioned rolled oats

½ cup natural peanut butter

¼ cup chia seeds

2 tablespoons pure maple syrup, divided

¼ teaspoon kosher salt

2 cups mixed berries

¼ cup chopped unsalted walnuts or almonds

1. In a medium mixing bowl, whisk together the milk, oats, peanut butter, chia seeds, 1 tablespoon of the maple syrup, and the salt until combined.

2. Divide the mixture among six small jars or airtight containers. Cover and refrigerate for 4 hours or overnight.

3. Before serving, top with the berries, nuts, and the remaining tablespoon of maple syrup.

4. Store the overnight oats in an airtight container in the refrigerator for up to 3 days.

Variation Tip: Swap ground flaxseed for the chia seeds. It may change the texture, but it will provide the same nutritional benefits. Top with apples or bananas instead of berries.

Cooking Tip: After you've whisked the ingredients together, let them sit for 10 minutes, then whisk them again. This will ensure that the ingredients are evenly distributed.

Nutrition Information (per serving): Calories 397; Total fat 19g; Saturated fat 3g; Cholesterol 3mg; Sodium 179mg; Carbs 42g; Fiber 9g; Sugar 15g; Protein 15g

RASPBERRY-HONEY PANCAKES

SERVES 4 / PREP TIME: 10 MINUTES / COOK TIME: 20 TO 25 MINUTES

Pancakes are the ultimate comfort food, and in this recipe, I've given them a healthy makeover without sacrificing the traditional pancake flavor and texture we all know and love. One trick to making fluffier pancakes is to choose finer, softer whole wheat pastry flour instead of regular whole wheat flour. Berries, a MIND diet superfood, are mixed into the batter, and the cooked pancakes are finished with peanut butter (for a protein boost) and a light drizzle of maple syrup.

3 tablespoons avocado oil or canola oil

5 tablespoons honey

1 large egg

1 tablespoon pure vanilla extract

1 cup milk

1½ cups whole wheat pastry flour or all-purpose flour

1½ teaspoons baking powder

½ teaspoon kosher salt

1 cup raspberries

Nonstick cooking spray

4 tablespoons natural peanut butter or almond butter

2 tablespoons pure maple syrup (optional)

1. In a large mixing bowl, use a hand mixer to beat the oil, honey, and egg until fluffy. Add the vanilla extract and milk, and beat until combined. Sift in the flour, baking powder, and salt. Beat until combined. Fold in the raspberries.

2. Place a large skillet over medium-high heat. Coat it with cooking spray. Working in batches, pour ¼ cup of the batter into the hot skillet and cook for 2 minutes per side, until set. Repeat with the remaining batter.

3. Spread the nut butter on the pancakes, and drizzle with maple syrup, if desired.

4. The pancakes can be prepped in advance and stored in a large sealed plastic bag or an airtight container for up to 4 days in the refrigerator or up to 2 months in the freezer. Reheat the pancakes in the microwave for 30 to 60 seconds or until heated through.

Variation Tip: Swap out the cow's milk for almond, coconut, or soy milk. Skip the step of folding the raspberries into the batter, and serve them on top instead.

Cooking Tip: To ensure that you get fluffy, lightly browned pancakes, let the pan heat up over medium-high heat before you add the batter.

Make It a Meal: Serve the pancakes with scrambled eggs or chicken or turkey sausage for a higher-protein meal.

Nutrition Information (per serving, 2 pancakes): Calories 459; Total fat 21g; Saturated fat 3g; Cholesterol 48mg; Sodium 422mg; Carbs 56g; Fiber 8g; Sugar 20g; Protein 13g

BANANA-NUT BREAKFAST PORRIDGE

SERVES 8 / PREP TIME: 10 MINUTES / COOK TIME: 30 TO 40 MINUTES

Porridge isn't just for the three bears, and it doesn't have to be made with just oats! In this version, I use farro, a type of wheat grain, because it is nutty and chewy. The added vanilla, brown sugar, and cinnamon make the house smell like Christmas. I like to serve it with walnuts or almonds and caramelized bananas for a boost of brain-healthy nutrients and potassium-rich sweetness.

2 cups farro

5 cups milk

¼ cup packed brown sugar

½ teaspoon pure vanilla extract

¼ teaspoon kosher salt

1 teaspoon ground cinnamon, divided

½ cup chopped unsalted walnuts or almonds

1 tablespoon avocado oil or canola oil

2 medium bananas, peeled and sliced

1. In a saucepan over medium heat, bring the farro and milk to a low simmer. Cook for 25 to 30 minutes, stirring frequently, until the farro is soft and most of the liquid has been absorbed. Stir in the brown sugar, vanilla, salt, and ½ teaspoon of the cinnamon.

2. Heat a dry skillet over medium-low heat. Add the nuts and toast, stirring constantly, for 30 to 60 seconds or until they are lightly browned. Remove the nuts from the skillet and set them aside.

3. Return the skillet to the stove over medium heat and add the oil. When the oil is hot, add the sliced bananas, sprinkle them with the remaining ½ teaspoon of cinnamon, and sauté for 1 to 2 minutes per side, until the bananas are browned and caramelized.

4. Serve the porridge with the caramelized bananas and toasted nuts.

5. Store the porridge in a microwaveable airtight container, and refrigerate for up to 4 days. Serve it cold or reheat it by microwaving on high for 1 to 3 minutes until heated through.

Variation Tip: Swap out the cow's milk for almond, coconut, or soy milk. Use apples instead of bananas.

Cooking Tip: Be careful not to burn the nuts when toasting them. The trick is to keep the heat at medium low, stir or shake the pan constantly, and only cook them until they are very lightly browned.

Nutrition Information (per serving): Calories 339; Total fat 8g; Saturated fat 1g; Cholesterol 3mg; Sodium 107mg; Carbs 57g; Fiber 6g; Sugar 18g; Protein 13g

MINI SPINACH AND POTATO FRITTATAS

MAKES 12 FRITTATA CUPS / PREP TIME: 10 TO 15 MINUTES / COOK TIME: 20 TO 30 MINUTES

Egg muffins are super trendy and popular, and for good reason. They can be made in advance and reheated for breakfast during the week, they can be loaded up with veggies and seasonings, and they are a great source of protein. This version features hash browns, spinach, roasted red peppers, and Italian seasonings, but you can customize them with whatever fillings you have on hand.

Nonstick cooking spray

1 tablespoon extra-virgin olive oil

3 cups baby spinach, roughly chopped

3 to 4 garlic cloves, minced

10 large eggs, beaten

2 cups frozen shredded or cubed potatoes, thawed

½ cup nonfat plain Greek yogurt

¼ cup chopped roasted red peppers

1¼ teaspoons kosher salt or sea salt

1 teaspoon Italian seasoning

¾ teaspoon onion powder

¼ teaspoon freshly ground black pepper

¼ teaspoon crushed red pepper flakes

1. Preheat the oven to 375°F. Coat a 12-cup muffin tin with cooking spray. Set aside.

2. Heat the olive oil in a large oven-safe nonstick or cast-iron skillet over medium heat. Add the spinach and garlic and sauté for 2 to 3 minutes, until the spinach is wilted. Remove from the heat.

3. In a large mixing bowl, stir together the eggs, potatoes, yogurt, roasted red peppers, salt, Italian seasoning, onion powder, black pepper, and red pepper flakes until thoroughly combined. Add the spinach mixture to the bowl and stir to combine.

4. Pour the egg mixture into the muffin tin wells, filling each about three-quarters of the way full. Bake for 20 to 22 minutes or until the frittatas are set.

5. Store the frittata cups in a microwaveable airtight container, and refrigerate for up to 5 days. Reheat them by microwaving on high for 1 to 3 minutes or until they are heated through.

Variation Tip: For a lower-fat frittata, use egg whites instead of whole eggs. Try kale or Swiss chard instead of spinach.

Cooking Tip: You can also make this recipe as a casserole. Simply coat a baking dish with cooking spray, pour the mixture into the pan, and bake at 375°F for 30 to 35 minutes, until set. Cut into squares and serve.

Nutrition Information (per serving, 1 frittata cup): Calories 97; Total fat 5g; Saturated fat 1g; Cholesterol 156mg; Sodium 189mg; Carbs 5g; Fiber 1g; Sugar 1g; Protein 7g

RAINBOW CHARD AND SWEET POTATO HASH

SERVES 4 / PREP TIME: 10 TO 15 MINUTES / COOK TIME: 20 TO 30 MINUTES

Rainbow chard is not only packed with nutrition—it's beautiful, too! You can use both the green leaves and the bright red stems in this hash, and its slightly bitter taste pairs perfectly with the sweet potatoes. This is served with sunny-side-up eggs to make a balanced meal.

3 tablespoons extra-virgin olive oil

1 large sweet potato, skin-on, diced

¼ medium sweet onion, diced

1 bunch rainbow chard (stalks and greens separated), chopped

2 to 3 garlic cloves, minced

¾ teaspoon kosher salt or sea salt, divided

½ teaspoon freshly ground black pepper, divided

¼ teaspoon crushed red pepper flakes

8 large eggs

1. Heat the olive oil in a large nonstick skillet over medium heat. Add the sweet potato, onion, and rainbow chard stalks and cook, stirring occasionally, for 15 to 20 minutes or until the potatoes are slightly tender.

2. Stir in the chard greens and garlic and cook for 2 to 3 more minutes, until the greens are wilted. Stir in ½ teaspoon of the salt, ¼ teaspoon of the black pepper, and the red pepper flakes.

3. Use a spatula to create eight wells in the hash. Crack an egg into each well, season with the remaining ¼ teaspoon salt and ¼ teaspoon black pepper, and place a lid on the skillet. Cook for 4 to 5 more minutes, until the egg whites are cooked through.

4. Store the hash in a microwaveable airtight container, and refrigerate for up to 5 days. Reheat it by microwaving on high for 1 to 3 minutes, until heated through.

Variation Tip: Use regular potatoes instead of sweet potatoes for a more savory hash. Try kale or spinach instead of rainbow chard.

Cooking Tip: If your pan is not large enough to cook all eight eggs in the hash, transfer the hash to plates and then cook the eggs in batches, as needed.

Nutrition Information (per serving): Calories 296; Total fat 20g; Saturated fat 5g; Cholesterol 372mg; Sodium 548mg; Carbs 15g; Fiber 3g; Sugar 4g; Protein 15g

SHAKSHUKA WITH POACHED EGGS

SERVES 4 / PREP TIME: 10 TO 15 MINUTES / COOK TIME: 20 TO 25 MINUTES

Shakshuka is a Middle Eastern dish consisting of eggs poached in a red pepper tomato sauce with spices like smoked paprika, cumin, and oregano. Not only is it loaded with flavor, but it also contains nutrients like lutein (from the tomatoes and eggs) that help keep your brain healthy. If you need to get another serving of greens into your day, add a handful of spinach or another dark leafy green. Serve it with whole-grain bread to soak up the sauce.

2 tablespoons extra-virgin olive oil

1 medium yellow onion, diced

1 large red bell pepper, seeded and diced

½ small jalapeño, seeded and minced

3 to 4 garlic cloves, minced

1 tablespoon smoked paprika

1 teaspoon ground cumin

1 teaspoon dried oregano

1¼ teaspoons kosher salt or sea salt, divided

½ teaspoon freshly ground black pepper, divided

1 (28-ounce) can no-salt-added crushed tomatoes

1 teaspoon granulated sugar (optional)

½ cup fresh cilantro leaves, chopped, divided

8 large eggs

1. Heat the olive oil in a large nonstick skillet over medium heat. Add the onion, bell pepper, and jalapeño and sauté for 3 to 4 minutes, until the vegetables are soft. Stir in the garlic, smoked paprika, cumin, oregano, 1 teaspoon of the salt, and ¼ teaspoon of the black pepper; sauté for 30 to 60 seconds, until fragrant.

2. Add the crushed tomatoes and bring the mixture to a simmer. Stir in the sugar, if using, and half of the cilantro.

3. Crack the eggs into the tomato sauce, about ½ inch apart, and sprinkle with the remaining salt and black pepper. Cover the pot and reduce the heat to medium low. Cook until the egg whites are set, 6 to 8 minutes. Sprinkle with the remaining chopped cilantro.

4. Store the shakshuka in microwaveable airtight containers, and refrigerate for up to 5 days. Reheat it by microwaving on high for 1 to 3 minutes, until heated through.

Variation Tip: If you don't have jalapeño, add a pinch of crushed red pepper flakes instead. For a boost of nutrients, add a handful of greens, such as spinach, kale, or Swiss chard, when sautéing the vegetables.

Cooking Tip: Adding a teaspoon of sugar is optional, but it helps balance the acidity of the tomato sauce.

Nutrition Information (per serving): Calories 328; Total fat 17g; Saturated fat 4g; Cholesterol 372mg; Sodium 548mg; Carbs 26g; Fiber 4g; Sugar 14g; Protein 18g

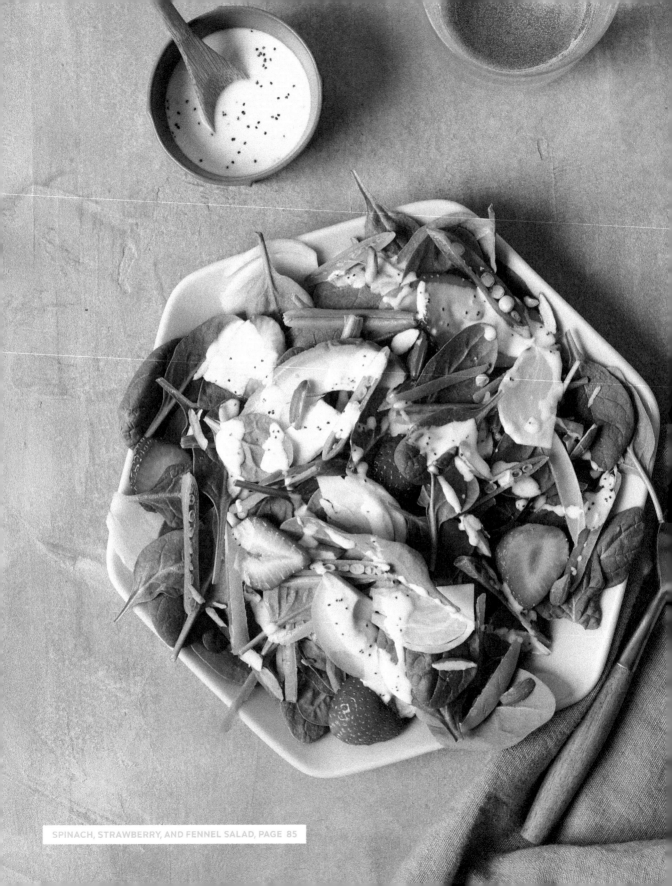

CHAPTER FIVE

Salads, Soups, and Sides

TRIPLE BERRY CHICKEN SALAD

SERVES 4 / PREP TIME: 15 MINUTES

Making your own salad dressing is simple—all you need is oil, vinegar, and seasonings, and you can customize it to pair nicely with your salad ingredients. In this case, I pair a dressing of extra-virgin olive oil, white wine vinegar, and honey with berries, chicken, nuts, and feta. You can add some cooked grains or chickpeas to make this an even higher-fiber salad.

For the dressing

2 tablespoons white wine vinegar

1 tablespoon honey

3 tablespoons extra-virgin olive oil

¼ teaspoon kosher salt or sea salt

⅛ teaspoon freshly ground black pepper

For the salad

5 to 6 cups spring mix

1 pound cooked chicken breast, sliced

1½ cups assorted fresh berries

¼ cup chopped unsalted walnuts or pecans

3 tablespoons crumbled feta cheese

To make the dressing

In a small bowl, whisk together the vinegar, honey, olive oil, salt, and black pepper. Cover and refrigerate.

To make the salad

1. Arrange the spring mix in four bowls. Evenly distribute the chicken, berries, nuts, and feta in each bowl. Before serving, drizzle with the dressing.

2. Store any undressed salad in an airtight container in the refrigerator for up to 3 days. Store the dressing in a small airtight container in the refrigerator for up to 5 days. Dress the salad just before serving.

Variation Tip: Try balsamic vinegar instead of white wine vinegar.

Cooking Tip: To cook the chicken breasts, heat 1 tablespoon of olive oil in a skillet over medium heat. Season the chicken with salt and black pepper, and cook for 3 to 5 minutes per side, until the chicken is browned and its internal temperature reaches 165°F. Let it cool before slicing.

Make It a Meal: Serve with a 3- to 4-inch piece of whole-grain baguette or add ¼ cup cooked grains (such as quinoa) to each salad.

Nutrition Information (per serving): Calories 406; Total fat 21g; Saturated fat 4g; Cholesterol 100mg; Sodium 272mg; Carbs 14g; Fiber 2g; Sugar 9g; Protein 38g

ROASTED BEET, ARUGULA, AND QUINOA SALAD

SERVES 6 / PREP TIME: 15 MINUTES / COOK TIME: 20 TO 25 MINUTES

Sweet, caramelized roasted beets paired with slightly bitter, crisp arugula and tangy, creamy goat cheese are a match made in heaven. This salad features those three ingredients, plus a handful of nutty quinoa, a delicious lemon vinaigrette, and crunchy sunflower seeds to make for a light—yet satisfying—meal.

For the dressing

Zest and juice of 1 medium lemon

3 tablespoons extra-virgin olive oil

1 tablespoon honey

¼ teaspoon kosher salt or sea salt

¼ teaspoon freshly ground black pepper

To make the dressing

In a small bowl, whisk together the lemon zest and juice, olive oil, honey, salt, and black pepper.

To make the salad

1. Preheat the oven to 400°F.

2. Place the beets on a baking sheet and coat them with the oil, then sprinkle with ¼ teaspoon of the salt and ¼ teaspoon of the black pepper. Roast for 20 to 25 minutes, until slightly fork tender. Remove from the oven and let cool.

3. Meanwhile, bring 2 cups of water to a boil in a medium saucepan. Add the quinoa and cook, stirring occasionally, until the water is absorbed, about 10 minutes. Remove the pan from the heat; set it aside to cool.

4. Assemble the salads by arranging the arugula, roasted beets, quinoa, shallots, sunflower seeds, and goat cheese, if using, on four plates. Drizzle with the dressing and serve immediately.

For the salad

4 medium beets, peeled and cubed

2 tablespoons avocado oil or canola oil

¾ teaspoon kosher salt, divided

½ teaspoon freshly ground black pepper, divided

1 cup quinoa, rinsed

2 cups fresh arugula

1 medium shallot, thinly sliced

¼ cup unsalted shelled sunflower seeds

2 tablespoons crumbled goat cheese (optional)

5. Store any undressed salad in an airtight container in the refrigerator for up to 3 days. Store the dressing in a small airtight container in the refrigerator for up to 5 days. Dress the salad just before serving.

Variation Tip: Try spinach or kale instead of arugula. Try farro, wheat berries, or another ancient grain instead of quinoa.

Cooking Tip: Cook the quinoa and other whole grains in unsalted broth instead of water for extra flavor.

Make It a Meal: Add cooked salmon, chicken, or turkey breast for a high-protein meal.

Nutrition Information (per serving): Calories 279; Total fat 14g; Saturated fat 2g; Cholesterol 0mg; Sodium 187mg; Carbs 29g; Fiber 4g; Sugar 8g; Protein 6g

CLASSIC TABBOULEH

SERVES 6 / PREP TIME: 15 MINUTES / COOK TIME: 15 TO 20 MINUTES

Bulgur is a type of wheat grain that is a traditional ingredient in this Middle Eastern salad. Unlike other grains, it doesn't require simmering on a stove; you simply pour boiling water over it and let it steam for about 15 minutes. Once it's cool, mix it with an entire bunch of chopped parsley, Roma tomatoes, cucumbers, extra-virgin olive oil, and fresh lemon zest and juice.

1 cup bulgur

2 cups boiling water

4 medium Roma tomatoes, diced

1 medium English cucumber, diced

2 cups fresh flat-leaf Italian parsley leaves, chopped

½ cup fresh mint leaves, chopped (optional)

6 tablespoons extra-virgin olive oil

Zest and juice of 1½ medium lemons

2 teaspoons kosher salt or sea salt

½ teaspoon freshly ground black pepper

1. Place the bulgur in a medium glass bowl. Pour the boiling water over the bulgur, stir, and cover with plastic wrap; let it stand for 15 to 20 minutes. Drain the bulgur of excess water, return it to the bowl, and set it aside to cool.

2. To the bowl, add the tomatoes, cucumber, parsley, mint (if using), olive oil, lemon zest and juice, salt, and black pepper; stir to combine. Taste and adjust the seasonings, if necessary. Refrigerate for at least 30 minutes before serving.

3. Store the tabbouleh in an airtight container in the refrigerator for up to 3 days.

Variation Tip: Although bulgur is the classic choice for tabbouleh, you could substitute another ancient grain, such as quinoa or farro. Try chopped cherry or grape tomatoes instead of Roma tomatoes.

Cooking Tip: Omit the lemon zest for a milder flavor.

Make It a Meal: Serve with cooked salmon, chicken, or turkey breast for a high-protein meal.

Nutrition Information (per serving): Calories 191; Total fat 14g; Saturated fat 2g; Cholesterol 0mg; Sodium 398mg; Carbs 14g;

SPINACH, STRAWBERRY, AND FENNEL SALAD

SERVES 4 / PREP TIME: 15 MINUTES

Fennel is an often-forgotten vegetable that tastes like anise, or black licorice. It pairs nicely in this salad with sweet strawberries and creamy avocado, served over a bed of spinach with a rich poppy seed dressing. Add cooked salmon to this salad for a boost of omega-3s and to make it a complete meal.

For the dressing

½ cup plain yogurt (not Greek)

2 tablespoons mayonnaise

2½ tablespoons honey or granulated sugar

2 tablespoons apple cider vinegar

Zest and juice of ½ medium lemon

1 tablespoon poppy seeds

¼ teaspoon kosher salt or sea salt

For the salad

6 cups baby spinach

2 cups fresh strawberries, hulled and sliced

2 medium avocados, sliced

1 small fennel bulb, thinly sliced

½ cup sugar snap peas, thinly sliced

¼ cup sliced unsalted almonds

To make the dressing

In a medium bowl, whisk together the yogurt, mayonnaise, honey or sugar, apple cider vinegar, lemon zest and juice, poppy seeds, and salt. Taste and adjust the seasonings, if necessary.

To make the salad

1. Arrange the spinach on four plates. Evenly distribute the strawberries, avocado, fennel, snap peas, and almonds. Drizzle with the dressing just before serving.

2. Store the undressed salad in an airtight container in the refrigerator for up to 3 days. Refrigerate the dressing in a separate container for up to 5 days. Dress the salad just before serving.

Variation Tip: Try walnuts or pecans instead of almonds. Try red wine vinegar instead of apple cider vinegar.

Cooking Tip: Save the fennel fronds (the dill-like tops of the stalk), chop them, and whisk them into the dressing for a stronger anise flavor.

Nutrition Information (per serving): Calories 308; Total fat 20g; Saturated fat 3g; Cholesterol 5mg; Sodium 212mg; Carbs 31g; Fiber 12g; Sugar 15g; Protein 8g

KALE AND CRISPY CHICKPEA CAESAR SALAD

SERVES 4 / PREP TIME: 15 MINUTES / COOK TIME: 30 TO 35 MINUTES

Caesar dressing is typically high in saturated fat, so I gave it a nutritional upgrade here by using extra-virgin olive oil as the base ingredient. It's bursting with flavor from fresh Parmesan, anchovies, garlic, lemon, and Worcestershire sauce, and it goes perfectly with a hearty green like kale. Instead of traditional croutons, roasted chickpeas add a healthy crunch.

For the crispy chickpeas

1 (15-ounce) can no-salt-added chickpeas, drained and rinsed

2 tablespoons extra-virgin olive oil

¼ teaspoon kosher salt or sea salt

For the Caesar dressing

¼ cup extra-virgin olive oil

2 tablespoons mayonnaise

2 tablespoons freshly grated Parmesan cheese

½ anchovy fillet, finely minced, or 1 teaspoon anchovy paste

2 garlic cloves, minced

Zest and juice of ½ medium lemon

2 teaspoons Worcestershire sauce

1 teaspoon granulated sugar

To make the crispy chickpeas

1. Preheat the oven to 425°F.

2. Lay paper towels out on a cutting board. Pour the chickpeas onto the paper towels and pat them dry. Transfer the chickpeas to a large mixing bowl. Add the olive oil and salt; toss to coat. Transfer the mixture to a baking sheet, and spread the chickpeas in one even layer. Roast in the oven for 30 to 35 minutes or until crispy, stirring halfway through. Remove the chickpeas from the oven and set them aside to cool.

To make the Caesar dressing

1. In the same bowl you used to season the chickpeas, whisk together the olive oil, mayonnaise, Parmesan, anchovy, garlic, lemon zest and juice, Worcestershire, sugar, salt, and black pepper. Taste and adjust the seasonings, if necessary.

2. Add the kale to the bowl and stir to thoroughly coat it with the dressing.

¼ teaspoon kosher salt or sea salt

½ teaspoon freshly ground black pepper

For the salad

1 large bunch lacinato kale, stemmed and chopped

¼ cup freshly grated Parmesan cheese

To assemble the salad

1. When ready to serve, distribute the dressed kale among four large bowls. Top each serving with crispy chickpeas and Parmesan cheese.

2. Store the kale salad in an airtight container in the refrigerator for up to 3 days. Store the chickpeas in an airtight container or a sealed plastic bag at room temperature for up to 7 days. Toss together just before serving.

Variation Tip: Try a few tablespoons of nutritional yeast instead of Parmesan cheese. Add spices, such as dried basil and oregano, to the chickpeas before roasting.

Cooking Tip: To achieve crispy chickpeas, be sure they are adequately dried before tossing them in oil and roasting them.

Nutrition Information (per serving): Calories 326; Total fat 29g; Saturated fat 5g; Cholesterol 16mg; Sodium 424mg; Carbs 12g; Fiber 2g; Sugar 8g; Protein 6g

PESTO PASTA FAGIOLI

SERVES 8 / PREP TIME: 15 TO 20 MINUTES / COOK TIME: 20 TO 25 MINUTES

Pasta fagioli is loaded with brain foods, such as olive oil, vegetables, dark leafy greens, beans, and whole grains. I added a scoop of pesto to give the soup richness and that classic basil flavor. The lemon juice adds an acidic note and is one of my tricks for reducing the amount of salt added to the dish without sacrificing flavor. Serve with crusty whole-grain bread.

2 tablespoons extra-virgin olive oil

1 medium yellow onion, minced

2 medium carrots, peeled and diced

2 medium stalks celery, diced

4 cups chopped spinach or kale leaves

3 to 4 garlic cloves, minced

1½ tablespoons Italian seasoning

1½ teaspoons kosher salt or sea salt

½ teaspoon freshly ground black pepper

2 tablespoons prepared pesto sauce

1 (15-ounce) can no-salt-added cannellini beans, drained and rinsed

1 (15-ounce) can no-salt-added dark red kidney beans, drained and rinsed

1. Heat the olive oil in a stockpot or Dutch oven over medium heat. Add the onion, carrots, and celery and sauté for 6 to 7 minutes or until the vegetables are soft. Add the spinach or kale, garlic, Italian seasoning, salt, and black pepper and sauté for 1 to 3 minutes, until the greens are wilted and the garlic is fragrant.

2. Stir in the pesto, cannellini beans, and kidney beans, then add the broth. Bring to a simmer, then stir in the pasta. Let the mixture simmer, stirring occasionally, until the pasta is cooked, about 10 minutes. Stir in the lemon juice. Taste and adjust the seasonings, if necessary. Serve the soup with freshly grated Parmesan cheese, if desired.

3. Store the soup in an airtight container in the refrigerator for up to 5 days. Reheat in the microwave on high for 2 to 3 minutes or until heated through.

7 to 8 cups unsalted
vegetable broth

**1 cup whole-grain small-
shaped pasta (such as
ditalini, elbow macaroni, or
orecchiette)**

Juice of ¼ medium lemon

2 tablespoons freshly grated
Parmesan cheese (optional)

Variation Tip: Omit the pasta or use gluten-free pasta for a gluten-free version. Add diced zucchini to the dish when you stir in the pasta for an extra dose of veggies.

Cooking Tip: The longer a soup sits, the more flavorful it becomes.

Nutrition Information (per serving): Calories 200; Total fat 6g; Saturated fat 0g; Cholesterol 2mg; Sodium 459mg; Carbs 25g; Fiber 8g; Sugar 6g; Protein 8g

THREE-BEAN AND VEGETABLE CHILI

SERVES 6 / PREP TIME: 15 TO 20 MINUTES / COOK TIME: 20 TO 25 MINUTES

Chili is the perfect meal for a cold winter day. This version has three types of beans, fire-roasted tomatoes, and lots of chili powder, making it filling and flavorful. You can add meat to this recipe, but I don't think you'll even miss it!

2 tablespoons extra-virgin olive oil

1 medium yellow onion, diced

1 medium red bell pepper, seeded and diced

1 medium green bell pepper, seeded and diced

3 to 4 garlic cloves, minced

2 tablespoons chili powder

2 teaspoons kosher salt or sea salt

1½ teaspoons ground cumin

1½ teaspoons dried oregano

½ teaspoon freshly ground black pepper

1 (15-ounce) can no-salt-added black beans, drained and rinsed

1 (15-ounce) can no-salt-added pinto beans, drained and rinsed

1. Heat the olive oil in a stockpot or Dutch oven over medium heat. Add the onion and bell peppers and sauté for 6 to 7 minutes, until the vegetables are soft. Add the garlic, chili powder, salt, cumin, oregano, and black pepper and sauté for 1 to 3 minutes, until the garlic and spices are fragrant.

2. Add the canned beans and diced tomatoes. Bring the mixture to a simmer and cook, stirring occasionally, for about 10 minutes. Taste and adjust the seasonings, if necessary. Serve the chili topped with shredded Cheddar cheese, if desired.

3. Store the soup in an airtight container in the refrigerator for up to 5 days. Reheat it in the microwave on high for 2 to 3 minutes or until heated through.

1 (15-ounce) can no-salt-added dark red kidney beans, drained and rinsed

2 (15-ounce) cans no-salt-added fire-roasted diced tomatoes

2 tablespoons shredded Cheddar cheese (optional)

Variation Tip: Add diced cooked chicken breast for a meat version. Add a can of diced green chiles and a small bag of frozen fire roasted corn kernels for a Mexican-style chili.

Cooking Tip: To use dried beans, soak them in water for at least 4 hours, rinse and drain them, and cook them in a pot of simmering water until tender.

Nutrition Information (per serving): Calories 284; Total fat 5g; Saturated fat 1g; Cholesterol 0mg; Sodium 385mg; Carbs 45g; Fiber 16g; Sugar 7g; Protein 14g

TOMATO-BASIL BISQUE

SERVES 6 / PREP TIME: 5 TO 10 MINUTES / COOK TIME: 15 TO 20 MINUTES

Tomato soup reminds me of being a kid, especially on snowy days. We'd always have it with grilled cheese sandwiches, of course. This is a grown-up version, as it calls for fresh basil, cayenne pepper, and just a bit of cream, but it's easy to make and comes together in less than 30 minutes. You'll never want to buy canned soup again after trying this recipe!

3 tablespoons extra-virgin olive oil

1 medium yellow onion, diced

3 to 4 garlic cloves, minced

1 tablespoon Italian seasoning

2½ teaspoons kosher salt or sea salt

½ teaspoon freshly ground black pepper

1 (28-ounce) can no-salt-added crushed tomatoes

2 cups unsalted vegetable broth

¼ cup fresh basil leaves

1 tablespoon balsamic vinegar

1. Heat the olive oil in a stockpot or Dutch oven over medium heat. Add the onion and sauté for 6 to 7 minutes, until soft. Add the garlic, Italian seasoning, salt, and pepper and sauté for 1 to 3 minutes, until the garlic and herbs are fragrant.

2. Add the crushed tomatoes and broth. Bring to a simmer and cook, stirring occasionally, for about 10 minutes.

3. Stir in the basil leaves. Use an immersion blender to purée the soup until it is very smooth.

4. Stir in the vinegar, sugar, cayenne, and cream or half-and-half. Taste and adjust the seasonings, if necessary. Serve with freshly grated Parmesan cheese, if desired.

1½ teaspoons granulated
sugar

¼ teaspoon cayenne pepper

3 tablespoons heavy cream
or half-and-half

2 tablespoons freshly grated
Parmesan cheese (optional)

5. Store the soup in an airtight container in the refrigerator for up to 5 days. Reheat it in the microwave on high for 2 to 3 minutes or until heated through.

Variation Tip: Skip the cream and Parmesan cheese to make the soup vegan. Use three roasted red bell peppers instead of the tomatoes to make roasted red pepper soup.

Cooking Tip: Use San Marzano tomatoes for a sweeter soup.

Nutrition Information (per serving): Calories 210; Total fat 10g; Saturated fat 3g; Cholesterol 10mg; Sodium 617mg; Carbs 19g; Fiber 5g; Sugar 17g; Protein 5g

ITALIAN WEDDING SOUP

SERVES 6 / PREP TIME: 15 TO 20 MINUTES / COOK TIME: 20 TO 25 MINUTES

This traditional soup, with its characteristic mini meatballs, may seem like it takes forever to make, but this recipe has a shortcut to save you time without sacrificing flavor. I use turkey or chicken Italian sausage and roll the filling into small balls, resembling meatballs. It requires fewer ingredients and provides the same delicious flavors you know and love.

1 tablespoon extra-virgin olive oil

1 pound uncooked Italian-style turkey or chicken sausage, casings removed

4 cups chopped spinach or kale leaves

3 to 4 garlic cloves, minced

¾ cup whole-grain orzo or acini de pepe pasta

4 cups unsalted chicken stock

1 to 2 cubes unsalted all-natural bouillon (optional)

¾ teaspoon kosher salt or sea salt

½ teaspoon freshly ground black pepper

2 large eggs

2 tablespoons freshly grated Parmesan cheese (optional)

1. Heat the olive oil in a stockpot or Dutch oven over medium heat. Form the sausage into ½-inch meatballs. Add the meatballs to the pot and sauté for 8 to 10 minutes, turning to lightly brown them on all sides. Add the spinach or kale and sauté for 2 to 3 minutes or until wilted. Stir in the garlic and pasta.

2. Add the stock and bring it to a simmer. Stir in the bouillon, if using, and salt and black pepper.

3. In a small bowl, whisk together the eggs and Parmesan cheese, if using. Use a spoon to create a whirlpool in the soup. As the liquid swirls, slowly pour in the egg mixture and simmer until the egg is set. Taste and adjust the seasonings, if necessary.

4. Store the soup in an airtight container in the refrigerator for up to 5 days. Reheat it in the microwave on high for 2 to 3 minutes or until heated through.

Variation Tip: Try Swiss chard or mustard greens for a bolder flavor. If you have a meatball recipe you love, use that instead of sausage.

Cooking Tip: Choose a bouillon that has no added salt or is labeled "low sodium."

Nutrition Information (per serving): Calories 280; Total fat 12g; Saturated fat 3g; Cholesterol 124mg; Sodium 600mg; Carbs 21g; Fiber 5g; Sugar 2g; Protein 21g

MAPLE BUTTERNUT SQUASH SOUP

SERVES 6 / PREP TIME: 15 TO 20 MINUTES / COOK TIME: 20 TO 30 MINUTES

The ginger, nutmeg, balsamic vinegar, coconut milk, and maple syrup are what make this soup really delicious. They complement the butternut squash without overpowering the flavor and texture of it, and the hint of cayenne pepper finishes it off on the perfect note. Be sure to add the spices to the pot before adding the liquid; sautéing releases the oils, making the spices more potent and flavorful.

3 tablespoons avocado oil or canola oil

½ medium yellow onion, diced

1 medium carrot, peeled and diced

2-inch piece fresh ginger, peeled and minced

2 teaspoons kosher salt or sea salt

1 teaspoon ground nutmeg

¼ teaspoon freshly ground black pepper

¼ teaspoon cayenne pepper

1 medium butternut squash, peeled, seeded, and cubed

3 cups unsalted vegetable broth

1 to 2 tablespoons balsamic vinegar

½ cup canned coconut milk

3 tablespoons pure maple syrup

1. Heat the oil in a stockpot or Dutch oven over medium heat. Add the onion and carrot and sauté for 3 to 4 minutes, until the vegetables are soft. Stir in the ginger, salt, nutmeg, black pepper, and cayenne. Add the cubed butternut squash.

2. Add the broth, bring it to a simmer, and cook for about 15 to 20 minutes, stirring occasionally, until the vegetables are very soft. Use an immersion blender to purée the soup until it is very smooth. (Alternatively, let the soup cool slightly, then transfer it to a blender and purée until smooth.) Stir in the balsamic vinegar, coconut milk, and maple syrup. Taste and adjust the seasonings, if necessary.

3. Store the soup in an airtight container in the refrigerator for up to 5 days. Reheat it in the microwave on high for 2 to 3 minutes or until heated through.

Variation Tip: Try freshly squeezed lime juice instead of balsamic vinegar. Swap out the squash for sweet potatoes.

Cooking Tip: If you're using a regular blender, remove the center piece on the lid and cover the entire lid with a kitchen towel. This allows some of the steam to escape so the top doesn't explode when blending a hot liquid. Start puréeing on low speed, and gradually increase the speed until the soup is silky smooth.

Nutrition Information (per serving): Calories 228; Total fat 11g; Saturated fat 4g; Cholesterol 0mg; Sodium 499mg; Carbs 32g; Fiber 4g; Sugar 15g; Protein 2g

ROASTED BALSAMIC ROOT VEGETABLES

SERVES 6 / PREP TIME: 15 TO 20 MINUTES / COOK TIME: 35 TO 45 MINUTES

As part of my weekly meal prep, I make a batch of roasted vegetables to be used as a side dish, made into soup, or used as the base for breakfast hash. You can use any root vegetable, as they all pair well with balsamic vinegar and olive oil. I roast them at 400°F until they are fork tender with a crispy exterior.

Nonstick cooking spray

2 medium sweet potatoes, peeled and cubed

2 medium parsnips, peeled and sliced

1 medium beet, peeled and cubed

1 medium red onion, thinly sliced

2 tablespoons balsamic vinegar

¼ cup avocado oil or canola oil

Leaves from 2 to 3 sprigs fresh thyme, chopped (optional)

1 teaspoon kosher salt or sea salt

½ teaspoon freshly ground black pepper

1. Preheat the oven to 400°F. Coat a baking sheet with cooking spray.

2. Place the sweet potatoes, parsnips, beet, and red onion on the baking sheet.

3. In a small bowl, whisk together the balsamic vinegar, oil, thyme (if using), salt, and black pepper until combined. Pour the mixture over the vegetables and toss to coat. Spread them out on the baking sheet in one even layer.

4. Roast the vegetables for 35 to 45 minutes, until they are tender and golden brown on the edges.

5. Store the roasted vegetables in an airtight container in the refrigerator for up to 5 days. Reheat them in the microwave on high for 2 to 3 minutes or until heated through.

Variation Tip: Try white balsamic vinegar for a milder flavor. After roasting, toss the vegetables with some freshly chopped basil.

Cooking Tip: To ensure that your veggies get crispy on the outside, do not overcrowd the pan.

Make It a Meal: Serve with over-easy eggs, cooked salmon, or roasted poultry.

Nutrition Information (per serving): Calories 227; Total fat 11g; Saturated fat 4g; Cholesterol 0mg; Sodium 312mg; Carbs 32g; Fiber 4g; Sugar 15g; Protein 2g

CINNAMON-ROASTED BUTTERNUT SQUASH

SERVES 4 / PREP TIME: 10 TO 15 MINUTES / COOK TIME: 40 TO 45 MINUTES

This recipe turns a classic fall-winter vegetable into candy! Squash is packed with beta carotene, lutein, and zeaxanthin, all of which are carotenoids that may be beneficial for brain health.

2 small butternut squash, halved and seeded

4 tablespoons avocado oil or canola oil

2½ teaspoons ground cinnamon, divided

½ teaspoon kosher salt or sea salt

¼ teaspoon cayenne pepper (optional)

2 tablespoons pure maple syrup or honey

1. Preheat the oven to 400°F.

2. Place the squash halves in a baking dish, cut-sides up.

3. In a small bowl, whisk together the oil, 2 teaspoons of cinnamon, salt, and cayenne, if using. Pour the mixture over the squash flesh.

4. Roast the squash until it is fork tender, 40 to 45 minutes. Remove it from the oven, drizzle with syrup or honey, and sprinkle with the remaining cinnamon before serving.

5. Store the squash in an airtight container in the refrigerator for up to 3 days. Reheat it in the microwave on high for 2 to 3 minutes or until heated through.

Variation Tip: Use pure maple syrup for a vegan version. Top with crunchy granola for a snack or breakfast.

Cooking Tip: Microwave the whole squash for 2 to 3 minutes to make slicing easier.

Make It a Meal: Serve with Moroccan-Style Chicken Tagine (page 170).

Nutrition Information (per serving, ½ squash): Calories 307; Total fat 14g; Saturated fat 2g; Cholesterol 0mg; Sodium 155mg; Carbs 48g; Fiber 7g; Sugar 14g; Protein 3g

GREEK-STYLE ORZO

SERVES 8 / PREP TIME: 10 TO 15 MINUTES / COOK TIME: 10 TO 15 MINUTES

Orzo is a rice-shaped pasta that is often used in Mediterranean dishes. This dish, filled with tomatoes, olives, and parsley, can be served on its own as a side dish or topped with cooked salmon or chicken for a complete meal. It features whole grains, olive oil, and tomatoes, all of which support brain health by providing B vitamins, heart-healthy fats, and antioxidants.

1 cup whole-grain orzo

Zest and juice of 1 medium lemon

1 tablespoon honey

¼ cup extra-virgin olive oil

2 garlic cloves, minced

2 teaspoons dried oregano

¾ teaspoon kosher salt or sea salt

¼ teaspoon freshly ground black pepper

1 pint cherry or grape tomatoes, quartered

⅓ cup pitted Kalamata olives

½ cup fresh flat-leaf Italian parsley leaves, chopped

¼ cup crumbled feta cheese

1. Cook the orzo according to the package directions. Drain and cool.

2. In a large bowl, whisk together the lemon zest and juice, honey, olive oil, garlic, oregano, salt, and black pepper. Fold in the orzo, tomatoes, olives, parsley, and feta cheese until combined.

3. Store the orzo in an airtight container in the refrigerator for up to 4 days.

Variation Tip: Use red wine vinegar instead of lemon juice, if desired. Try an ancient grain, such as quinoa or farro, instead of pasta.

Cooking Tip: If you cannot find whole-grain orzo, choose regular orzo or another whole-grain small-shaped pasta.

Make It a Meal: Serve with cooked salmon, chicken, or turkey breast for a high-protein meal.

Nutrition Information (per serving): Calories 186; Total fat 10g; Saturated fat 2g; Cholesterol 4mg; Sodium 314mg; Carbs 21g; Fiber 4g; Sugar 4g; Protein 4g

CLASSIC RATATOUILLE

SERVES 6 / PREP TIME: 20 TO 25 MINUTES / COOK TIME: 20 TO 30 MINUTES

Ratatouille is a classic French Provençal dish of stewed eggplant, zucchini, tomatoes, bell pepper, and basil. The olive oil gives it richness, and parsley adds color and freshness. Eggplant has a high water content, and sprinkling it with salt will draw out that moisture; be sure to pat it dry before adding it to the pot with the other ingredients.

1 large eggplant, peeled and cubed

2½ teaspoons kosher salt or sea salt, divided

¼ cup extra-virgin olive oil

1 large zucchini, halved lengthwise and sliced into half-moons

1 medium yellow onion, diced

1 medium red bell pepper, seeded and diced

2 pints cherry or grape tomatoes, cut in half, divided

4 garlic cloves, minced

2 teaspoons Italian seasoning

½ teaspoon freshly ground black pepper

⅛ teaspoon crushed red pepper flakes

1. Place the eggplant on a paper towel–lined plate, sprinkle with ¼ teaspoon salt, and toss well. Let it sit for 10 minutes, then pat the eggplant dry with a paper towel.

2. Heat the olive oil in a large saucepan or Dutch oven over medium heat. Sauté the eggplant for 7 to 8 minutes, stirring occasionally, until lightly browned. Add the zucchini, onion, bell pepper, and half of the tomatoes and cook for 5 to 6 minutes, stirring occasionally, until the vegetables are soft.

3. Stir in the garlic, Italian seasoning, the remaining 2¼ teaspoons salt, black pepper, and red pepper flakes. Stir in the basil, parsley, sugar, and remaining tomatoes and simmer for 4 to 5 more minutes. Taste and adjust the seasonings, if necessary.

4. Store the ratatouille in an airtight container in the refrigerator for up to 5 days. Reheat it in the microwave on high for 2 to 3 minutes or until heated through.

½ cup fresh basil, roughly chopped

¼ cup fresh flat-leaf Italian parsley leaves, chopped

1 teaspoon granulated sugar

Variation Tip: Substitute the eggplant with 2 additional zucchinis and/or summer squash, depending on the season. Use a few tablespoons of dried basil if fresh is not available.

Cooking Tip: If you have them on hand, add a pinch of dried marjoram and fennel.

Make It a Meal: Serve with Turkey-Zucchini Meat Loaf (page 176).

Nutrition Information (per serving): Calories 146; Total fat 10g; Saturated fat 1g; Cholesterol 0mg; Sodium 481mg; Carbs 14g; Fiber 5g; Sugar 9g; Protein 3g

CRISPY BAKED ARTICHOKE HEARTS

SERVES 4 / PREP TIME: 15 TO 20 MINUTES / COOK TIME: 15 TO 20 MINUTES

Fresh artichoke hearts can be a bit cumbersome to work with, but, lucky for us, canned and jarred artichokes are just as delicious—and so much easier! Artichokes are rich in folate, a B vitamin, and are also packed with fiber. I like to add them to salads, mix them into grain bowls, and, in this case, bread them and bake them until they're super crispy. These work well as a snack or an appetizer.

For the dipping oil

4 tablespoons extra-virgin olive oil

1 tablespoon balsamic vinegar

⅛ teaspoon kosher salt or sea salt

For the artichoke hearts

Nonstick cooking spray

1 (14.5-ounce) jar marinated artichoke hearts

¼ cup all-purpose flour

2 large eggs, beaten

¾ cup panko breadcrumbs

1 teaspoon kosher salt or sea salt

½ teaspoon freshly ground black pepper

¼ teaspoon crushed red pepper flakes

To make the dipping oil

In a small bowl, whisk together the olive oil, balsamic vinegar, and salt. Set aside.

To make the artichoke hearts

1. Preheat the oven to 425°F. Place a wire rack in a baking sheet, and coat it with cooking spray.

2. Drain the artichoke hearts, then transfer them to a plate lined with paper towels; thoroughly pat them dry.

3. Set up three bowls: one with flour, one with eggs, and one with breadcrumbs. Evenly distribute and stir the salt, black pepper, and crushed red pepper flakes in each bowl. Dip each artichoke heart into the flour, then the egg, and then the breadcrumbs. Place the breaded artichokes on the prepared rack and spritz them with cooking spray.

4. Bake for 15 to 20 minutes or until the artichokes are lightly browned and crispy. Serve with the dipping oil.

5. Store the baked artichoke hearts in an airtight container in the refrigerator for up to 4 days. To reheat, broil them on low for 3 to 4 minutes or until crispy and heated through. Make the dipping oil fresh as needed.

Variation Tip: Use gluten-free breadcrumbs for a gluten-free version. Skip the crushed red pepper flakes for a mild version.

Cooking Tip: Spritzing the coated artichoke hearts with cooking spray and baking them on a wire rack, versus directly on the pan, assures a crispy exterior.

Nutrition Information (per serving): Calories 131; Total fat 5g; Saturated fat 1g; Cholesterol 93mg; Sodium 370mg; Carbs 16g; Fiber 2g; Sugar 1g; Protein 5g

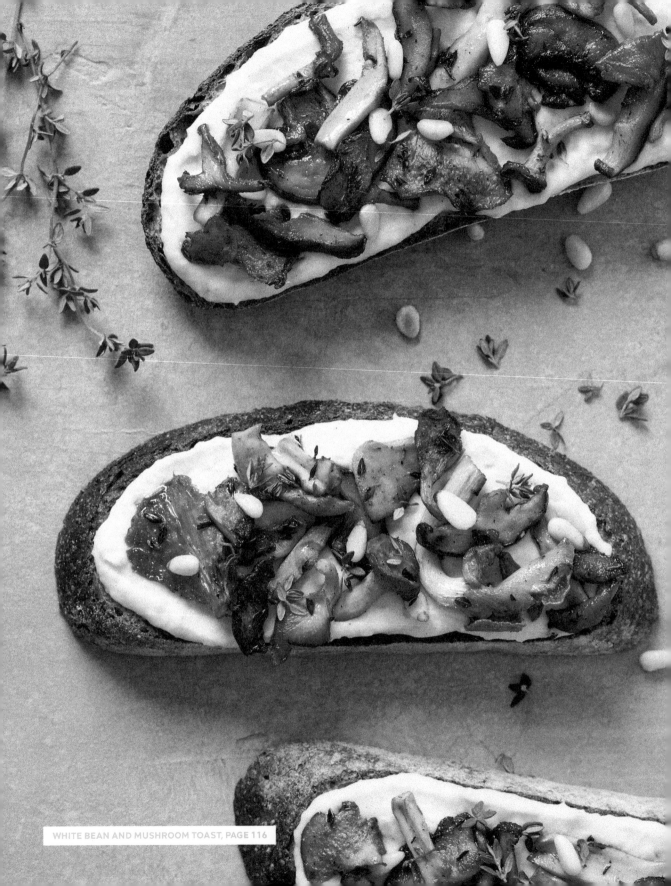

WHITE BEAN AND MUSHROOM TOAST, PAGE 116

Vegetarian Mains

BLACK BEAN NACHOS

SERVES 6 / PREP TIME: 20 TO 25 MINUTES / COOK TIME: 15 TO 20 MINUTES

Everyone loves nacho night! In this veggie variation of the party classic, fiber- and protein-rich beans are simmered in homemade taco seasoning and served on a bed of crispy tortilla chips with avocado, salsa, cilantro, and Greek yogurt. If you want to add meat, you can cook the beans with lean ground chicken, turkey, or beef.

For the black beans

1 tablespoon avocado oil or canola oil

2 tablespoons chili powder

1 teaspoon onion powder

1 teaspoon garlic powder

1 teaspoon ground cumin

1 teaspoon smoked paprika

1 teaspoon kosher salt or sea salt

½ teaspoon freshly ground black pepper

2 (15-ounce) cans no-salt-added black beans, drained and rinsed

For the nachos

6 ounces tortilla chips

2 medium ripe avocados, pitted and diced

1 cup salsa

1 cup fresh cilantro leaves, chopped

½ cup plain Greek yogurt

To make the black beans

1. Heat the oil in a large skillet over medium heat.

2. In a small bowl, whisk together the chili powder, onion powder, garlic powder, cumin, smoked paprika, salt, and black pepper. Add the spice mixture to the skillet and sauté for 30 to 60 seconds, until fragrant.

3. Add the beans and ¼ cup of water. Bring the mixture to a simmer and cook, stirring occasionally, for about 5 minutes or until thickened. Use a potato masher to gently mash some of the beans.

To make the nachos

1. Arrange the tortilla chips on six plates. Top with the black beans, avocado, salsa, cilantro, and Greek yogurt. Serve immediately.

2. Store the chips, black bean mixture and toppings in separate airtight containers. Refrigerate the black bean mixture and toppings for up to 4 days. Reheat the black bean mixture by microwaving on high for 1 to 3 minutes, until heated through. Assemble nachos just before serving.

Variation Tip: Skip the Greek yogurt for vegan nachos. Try pinto beans instead of black beans. To save time, use a prepackaged low-salt taco seasoning instead of the individual spices in the recipe. Melt a little shredded cheese on top of the black bean mixture.

Nutrition Information (per serving): Calories 487; Total fat 20g; Saturated fat 3g; Cholesterol 1mg; Sodium 327mg; Carbs 65g; Fiber 12g; Sugar 8g; Protein 14g

BAKED CHICKPEA AND SPINACH FALAFEL

SERVES 4 / PREP TIME: 10 TO 15 MINUTES / CHILLING TIME: 30 MINUTES
/ COOK TIME: 15 TO 20 MINUTES

This version of falafel is baked, not fried, and is loaded with chickpeas, spinach, lemon, fresh herbs, and garlic. You can eat it as is, or you can serve it in pita bread as a sandwich. The chickpeas provide B vitamins, and adding spinach gives the falafel a boost of vitamin E and folate, which support brain health.

1 (15-ounce) can no-salt-added chickpeas, drained and rinsed

2 cups baby spinach

⅔ cup panko breadcrumbs

½ cup fresh mixed herb leaves (such as parsley, cilantro, and dill)

½ **medium yellow onion, roughly chopped**

3 to 4 garlic cloves, peeled

Zest and juice of ½ medium lemon

1½ **tablespoons extra-virgin olive oil**

1 teaspoon kosher salt or sea salt

½ teaspoon freshly ground black pepper

½ teaspoon dried oregano

¼ teaspoon crushed red pepper flakes

Nonstick cooking spray

1. Place the chickpeas, spinach, breadcrumbs, herbs, onion, garlic, lemon zest and juice, olive oil, salt, black pepper, oregano, and red pepper flakes in the bowl of a food processor. Process until a smooth paste forms. Cover and refrigerate for at least 30 minutes.

2. Preheat the oven to 400°F. Fit a baking sheet with a wire rack, and coat it with cooking spray.

3. Form the mixture into 12 (2-inch) balls, and place them on the prepared rack. Bake for 15 to 20 minutes, until the outsides are slightly crispy.

4. Store the falafel in an airtight container in the refrigerator for up to 4 days. Reheat them by microwaving on high for 1 to 3 minutes, until heated through.

Variation Tip: Use any white bean, like cannellini or great northern beans. Substitute black beans instead of chickpeas, lime juice instead of lemon juice, and add 1 tablespoon of chili powder for Mexican-style falafel.

Cooking Tip: Spritz the falafel balls with cooking spray before baking for an extra crispy exterior.

Nutrition Information (per serving, 3 falafel balls):
Calories 152; Total fat 1g; Saturated fat 0g; Cholesterol 0mg;
Sodium 50mg; Carbs 17g; Fiber 6g; Sugar 1g; Protein 7g

CHICKPEA COCONUT CURRY

SERVES 6 / PREP TIME: 10 TO 15 MINUTES / COOK TIME: 20 TO 25 MINUTES

This is quite possibly the easiest—yet most delicious—curry recipe! I love that it's mostly made from pantry ingredients, so if you're in a rush or don't have many fresh groceries, you can still whip this up and enjoy a balanced meal. The coconut milk, peanut butter, ginger, and lime give the dish amazing flavor and texture. Garam masala is an Indian spice mixture that typically contains coriander, cinnamon, cumin, cardamom, black pepper, cloves, and nutmeg; it can be found in the spice aisle at the grocery store.

2 tablespoons extra-virgin olive oil

1 medium yellow onion, diced

3 cups chopped spinach, kale, or chard leaves

3 to 4 garlic cloves, minced

1-inch piece fresh ginger, peeled and minced

2 tablespoons garam masala

2 teaspoons kosher salt or sea salt

½ teaspoon freshly ground black pepper

¼ teaspoon cayenne pepper

2 (15-ounce) cans no-salt-added chickpeas, drained and rinsed

1 (15-ounce) can no-salt-added petite diced tomatoes, drained

1. In a large Dutch oven or stockpot, heat the olive oil over medium heat. Add the onion and sauté for 4 to 5 minutes, until soft. Stir in the greens, garlic, and ginger and sauté for 2 to 3 minutes or until the greens are wilted. Stir in the garam masala, salt, black pepper, and cayenne. Stir in the chickpeas, diced tomatoes, and vegetable broth and increase the heat to medium high. Simmer for about 10 to 15 minutes.

2. Remove the pot from the heat and stir in the coconut milk, peanut butter, lime zest and juice, honey, and half of the cilantro. Taste and adjust the seasonings, if necessary. Serve the curry over quinoa, topped with cashews and the remaining chopped cilantro.

3. Store the curry in an airtight container in the refrigerator for up to 4 days. Reheat it by microwaving on high for 2 to 3 minutes or until heated through.

½ to 1 cup unsalted vegetable broth

¾ cup canned coconut milk

2 tablespoons natural peanut butter

Zest and juice of 1 medium lime

1½ tablespoons honey

½ cup fresh cilantro leaves, chopped, divided

2 cups cooked quinoa

½ cup chopped cashews

Variation Tip: Add cooked chicken breast to make a meat version. Try this dish with lentils instead of chickpeas. Substitute brown rice for quinoa.

Cooking Tip: Keep a container of no-salt-added instant bouillon on hand in case you run out of stock or broth. Simply follow the directions on the back of the container to make your own.

Nutrition Information (per serving): Calories 403; Total fat 18g; Saturated fat 6g; Cholesterol 0mg; Sodium 525mg; Carbs 44g; Fiber 11g; Sugar 10g; Protein 14g

GARLICKY WHITE BEAN CASSOULET

SERVES 4 / PREP TIME: 10 TO 15 MINUTES / COOK TIME: 20 TO 25 MINUTES

This stovetop casserole reminds me of something I would've eaten as a kid. It's wholesome, hearty, and filling, and also super affordable. It's another dish that uses mainly pantry ingredients, but it's packed with flavor and nutrition. The Parmesan and panko crispy topping takes it from good to *great*.

4 tablespoons extra-virgin olive oil, divided

½ medium yellow onion, diced

5 to 6 garlic cloves, minced

Leaves from 1 sprig fresh rosemary, chopped

Leaves from 2 sprigs fresh thyme, chopped

2 (15-ounce) cans no-salt-added cannellini or great northern beans, drained and rinsed

1 cup unsalted vegetable broth

1 teaspoon kosher salt or sea salt

½ teaspoon freshly ground black pepper

1. In a large Dutch oven, heat 2 tablespoons of the olive oil over medium heat. Add the onion and sauté for 4 to 5 minutes, until soft. Add the garlic, rosemary, and thyme and sauté for 30 to 60 seconds or until fragrant. Add the beans, broth, salt, black pepper, and red pepper flakes and simmer for about 10 to 15 minutes, until thickened. Stir in the lemon zest and juice.

2. Preheat the broiler.

3. In a small bowl, whisk together the remaining 2 tablespoons of olive oil, the panko breadcrumbs, and the Parmesan cheese. Spoon the topping over the stew, transfer the Dutch oven to the oven, and broil for 3 to 4 minutes or until the topping is lightly browned.

¼ teaspoon crushed red pepper flakes

Zest and juice of ½ medium lemon

½ cup panko breadcrumbs

2 tablespoons freshly grated Parmesan cheese

4. Store the cassoulet in airtight containers in the refrigerator for up to 4 days. Reheat it by microwaving on high for 2 to 3 minutes or until heated through.

Variation Tip: To make this dish vegan, swap out the Parmesan cheese for nutritional yeast. Add chicken or turkey breast to make a meat version.

Cooking Tip: Swap in dried rosemary and thyme for the fresh, but use half the amount.

Nutrition Information (per serving): Calories 364; Total fat 15g; Saturated fat 2g; Cholesterol 3mg; Sodium 496mg; Carbs 42g; Fiber 12g; Sugar 4g; Protein 13g

WHITE BEAN AND MUSHROOM TOAST

SERVES 6 / PREP TIME: 10 TO 15 MINUTES / COOK TIME: 5 TO 10 MINUTES

Talk about a quick meal! This is the ultimate meal prep recipe, because all you have to do is make a batch of white bean spread, sauté some mushrooms, toast some whole-grain bread, and assemble. These are loaded with healthy brain foods, and they provide a burst of garlic, lemon, and thyme flavors to keep you coming back for more.

For the mushrooms

2 tablespoons extra-virgin olive oil

3 cups sliced mushrooms

Leaves from 2 sprigs fresh thyme, chopped

½ teaspoon kosher salt or sea salt

¼ teaspoon freshly ground black pepper

For the bean spread

1 (15-ounce) can no-salt-added cannellini or great northern beans, drained and rinsed

2 to 3 garlic cloves, minced

Zest and juice of ½ medium lemon

¾ teaspoon kosher salt or sea salt

To make the mushrooms

In a medium skillet, heat the olive oil over medium heat. Add the mushrooms and sauté for 5 to 6 minutes, stirring occasionally, until soft and browned. Stir in the thyme, salt, and black pepper. Remove the skillet from the heat.

To make the bean spread

Meanwhile, place the beans, garlic, lemon zest and juice, salt, black pepper, red pepper flakes, and olive oil in a food processor and process until smooth, stopping to scrape the sides of the bowl as needed. Taste and adjust the seasonings, if necessary.

To make the toast

1. Heat a small skillet over medium-low heat. Add the pine nuts and toast for 30 to 60 seconds or until fragrant, shaking the pan to keep them from burning. Transfer to a bowl and set aside.

2. Spread the bean spread on the toast, top with sautéed mushrooms, and sprinkle with toasted pine nuts.

¼ teaspoon freshly ground black pepper

⅛ teaspoon crushed red pepper flakes

¼ **cup extra-virgin olive oil**

For the toast

2 tablespoons pine nuts

6 slices whole-grain bread, toasted

3. Store the bean spread and mushrooms separately in airtight containers in the refrigerator up to 4 days. Serve leftovers cold or reheat the mushrooms by microwaving them on high for 30 to 60 seconds or until heated through.

Variation Tip: Try walnuts or pepitas instead of pine nuts. Add about ¼ cup tahini (sesame seed paste) to the bean spread to turn it into hummus. Make an extra batch for snacks!

Cooking Tip: If you're making this for multiple people, turn on the broiler and place several slices of bread on a baking sheet. Toast on each side for just a few minutes until browned and crisp.

Nutrition Information (per serving, 1 toast): Calories 335; Total fat 18g; Saturated fat 2g; Cholesterol 0mg; Sodium 279mg; Carbs 37g; Fiber 10g; Sugar 6g; Protein 9g

ZUCCHINI-LENTIL FRITTERS

SERVES 6 / PREP TIME: 10 TO 15 MINUTES / COOK TIME: 10 TO 15 MINUTES

Pretty much any vegetable, herb, and seasoning can go in fritter batter. In this instance, the fritters are made of zucchini, lentils, parsley, dill, lemon, and Dijon mustard, mixed together with flour and baking powder, and then lightly fried in olive oil. They can serve as a meal, side dish, or appetizer.

1 cup cooked green or red lentils

2 medium zucchini, grated

¼ medium yellow onion, minced

¼ cup fresh flat-leaf Italian parsley leaves, chopped

2 tablespoons chopped fresh dill

Zest and juice of ½ medium lemon

1 tablespoon Dijon mustard

½ cup all-purpose flour

2 large eggs

1 teaspoon baking powder

1 teaspoon kosher salt or sea salt

½ teaspoon freshly ground black pepper

¼ cup extra-virgin olive oil

1. Place the cooked lentils in a large bowl and lightly mash them with the back of a fork. Add the zucchini, onion, parsley, dill, lemon zest and juice, Dijon, flour, eggs, baking powder, salt, and black pepper. Stir until thoroughly combined.

2. Heat the olive oil in a large skillet over medium heat. Working in batches, spoon 2 tablespoons of batter into the hot oil for each fritter. Cook for 2 to 3 minutes, until browned and crispy, then flip and cook for another 1 to 2 minutes. Transfer the fritters to a paper towel–lined plate to dry.

3. Store the fritters in an airtight container in the refrigerator for up to 4 days. Reheat them in the microwave on high for 1 to 3 minutes or until heated through.

Variation Tip: Try summer squash instead of zucchini. Try making the fritters without lentils—just replace the beans with another cup of grated zucchini.

Cooking Tip: To save time, use canned lentils; simply rinse, drain, and dry them before adding them to the batter.

Make It a Meal: Serve alongside Honey Mustard Grilled Salmon (page 152).

Nutrition Information (per serving, 2 fritters): Calories 209; Total fat 12g; Saturated fat 2g; Cholesterol 62mg; Sodium 408mg; Carbs 19g; Fiber 5g; Sugar 2g; Protein 8g

KUNG PAO TOFU STIR-FRY

SERVES 6 / PREP TIME: 10 TO 15 MINUTES / COOK TIME: 15 TO 20 MINUTES

You can prep the tofu, kung pao sauce, vegetables, and rice in advance so this stir-fry comes together easier on a busy weeknight. Just toss it together in a hot skillet, and in minutes you'll have a flavorful takeout-inspired dish that is balanced, nutritious, and plant-based.

1 pound extra-firm tofu

For the sauce

¼ cup unsalted vegetable broth

2 teaspoons cornstarch

2 tablespoons low-sodium soy sauce

1 tablespoon rice wine vinegar

1 to 2 tablespoons granulated sugar

2 dried Thai chiles, crushed, or ½ teaspoon crushed red pepper flakes

1 teaspoon sesame oil

2 garlic cloves, minced

1-inch piece fresh ginger, peeled and minced

To prepare the tofu

Remove the block of tofu from its package and place it on a plate lined with a clean kitchen towel. Place another clean kitchen towel on top of the tofu, and weigh it down with a heavy pot. Let the tofu sit for 10 to 15 minutes, changing the towels if they become soaked. Remove the pot and towels, and cut the tofu into 1-inch cubes.

To make the sauce

In a small bowl, whisk together the broth and cornstarch until dissolved. Whisk in the soy sauce, vinegar, honey or sugar, crushed chiles, sesame oil, garlic, and ginger until combined. Set aside.

To make the stir-fry

1. Heat a large skillet over medium-low heat. Add the peanuts and toast for about 30 to 60 minutes, stirring constantly. Transfer them to a plate and set aside.

2. In the same skillet, heat the oil over medium-high heat. Add the tofu pieces, season with salt and black pepper, and sauté for 4 to 5 minutes, turning them with tongs to brown all sides. Add the red bell pepper and sauté for 2 to 3 minutes or until slightly softened. Add the sauce and let the entire mixture simmer for 1 to 2 minutes, until the sauce is thickened.

For the stir-fry

½ cup chopped unsalted peanuts

3 tablespoons avocado oil or canola oil

½ teaspoon kosher salt or sea salt

¼ teaspoon freshly ground black pepper

1 medium red bell pepper, seeded and chopped

2½ cups cooked brown rice

3 green onions, thinly sliced

3. Divide the brown rice among six bowls and top with the tofu stir-fry. Sprinkle with toasted peanuts and green onion.

4. Store the stir-fry in an airtight container in the refrigerator for up to 4 days. Reheat it in the microwave on high for 1 to 3 minutes or until heated through.

Variation Tip: Swap tofu for chicken, shrimp, or flank steak. Use any color bell pepper.

Cooking Tip: Batch prep garlic and ginger by placing several peeled cloves/pieces in a mini food processor and pulsing until they are minced. Store it in an airtight container in the fridge or freezer.

Nutrition Information (per serving): Calories 332; Total fat 18g; Saturated fat 2g; Cholesterol 0mg; Sodium 337mg; Carbs 31g; Fiber 4g; Sugar 6g; Protein 13g

GRILLED TOFU WITH PEACH-CUCUMBER SALSA

SERVES 4 / PREP TIME: 10 TO 15 MINUTES / COOK TIME: 20 TO 25 MINUTES

Grilling the tofu on medium-low heat helps create a crispy exterior, and the chili powder, cumin, and smoked paprika spice rub provides a deliciously spicy contrast to the light and refreshing cucumber-peach salsa. Serve it with cooked rice or another grain for a higher-fiber meal.

1 pound extra-firm tofu

For the salsa

1 medium English cucumber, diced

2 medium peaches, pitted and diced

¼ medium red onion, finely diced

½ medium jalapeño, seeded and finely diced

½ cup fresh cilantro leaves, chopped

Zest and juice of 1 medium lime

¼ teaspoon kosher salt or sea salt

To prepare the tofu

Remove the block of tofu from its package and place it on a plate lined with a clean kitchen towel. Place another clean kitchen towel on top of the tofu, and weigh it down with a heavy pot. Let the tofu sit for 10 to 15 minutes, changing the towels if they become soaked.

To make the salsa

In a medium glass bowl, mix together the cucumber, peaches, onion, jalapeño, cilantro, lime zest and juice, and salt. Cover and refrigerate.

To make the tofu

1. Heat a grill or grill pan over medium-low heat.

2. Cut the tofu into four squares. Rub the tofu pieces with oil. In a small bowl, whisk together the chili powder, cumin, smoked paprika, and salt. Dredge the oiled tofu pieces in the spice mixture. Place them on the grill and cook for 8 to 10 minutes per side, until the exterior is browned and the edges are crispy.

For the tofu

1 tablespoon avocado oil or canola oil

1 tablespoon chili powder

2 teaspoons ground cumin

1 teaspoon smoked paprika

½ teaspoon kosher salt or sea salt

3. Serve the tofu with a scoop of peach-cucumber salsa.

4. Store the tofu in an airtight container in the refrigerator for up to 4 days. Reheat it in the microwave on high for 1 to 3 minutes or until heated through. Refrigerate the salsa in a separate airtight container for up to 3 days.

Variation Tip: Try mango or pineapple in the salsa instead of peaches. Use this same spice rub on chicken breast to make a meat version.

Cooking Tip: Be sure the tofu is very dry; otherwise, it's difficult to achieve a crispy exterior when cooking.

Nutrition Information (per serving): Calories 193; Total fat 9g; Saturated fat 1g; Cholesterol 0mg; Sodium 289mg; Carbs 17g; Fiber 4g; Sugar 8g; Protein 12g

RIGATONI WITH BROCCOLI PESTO

SERVES 6 / PREP TIME: 10 TO 15 MINUTES / COOK TIME: 20 TO 25 MINUTES

Pesto is made with fresh basil, pine nuts, Parmesan, garlic, olive oil, salt, and black pepper. This version also includes several cups of broccoli to make a simple veggie-packed sauce that's delicious tossed with pasta. Finish it off with a handful of chopped herbs, and add a cooked fillet of salmon to make it a higher-protein meal.

8 ounces whole-grain rigatoni (or other whole-grain shaped pasta)

5 cups broccoli florets, cooked and cooled

¼ cup fresh basil leaves

¼ cup freshly grated Parmesan cheese, divided

¼ cup unsalted nuts (pine nuts, walnut pieces, chopped almonds, or pepitas)

Zest and juice of 1 medium lemon

3 to 4 garlic cloves, peeled

1¼ teaspoons kosher salt or sea salt

¼ teaspoon freshly ground black pepper

½ cup plus 2 tablespoons extra-virgin olive oil, plus more as needed

¼ cup fresh flat-leaf Italian parsley leaves, chopped

1. Bring a pot of water to a boil. Cook the pasta according to the package directions, to al dente. Reserve ½ cup of the pasta water, then drain the pasta.

2. In a food processor, pulse the broccoli florets until they are reduced to small chunks. Add the basil, 2 tablespoons of the Parmesan cheese, the nuts, lemon zest and juice, garlic, salt, and black pepper. Process on low, and with the motor running, drizzle in ½ cup of the olive oil; process until the mixture is creamy. Taste and adjust the seasonings, if necessary.

3. Pour the reserved pasta water into the same pot you used for cooking the pasta, and bring it to a simmer over medium heat. Add the broccoli pesto, bring it to a simmer, then reduce the heat to low and stir the sauce until it thickens. Fold in the pasta until combined.

4. Serve the pasta topped with the remaining Parmesan cheese, the remaining 2 tablespoons of olive oil, and the chopped parsley.

5. Store the pasta in an airtight container in the refrigerator for up to 4 days. Reheat it in the microwave on high for 1 to 3 minutes or until heated through, or enjoy it cold.

Variation Tip: Use any shape of whole-grain pasta (penne, bow ties, fusilli). Add a handful of spinach to the pesto for a boost of brain-healthy greens.

Cooking Tip: Al dente means "to the tooth." The pasta should have a bit of a bite but shouldn't be chewy.

Nutrition Information (per serving): Calories 388; Total fat 28g; Saturated fat 4g; Cholesterol 4mg; Sodium 324mg; Carbs 32g; Fiber 5g; Sugar 2g; Protein 8g

ASPARAGUS FARRO RISOTTO

SERVES 8 / PREP TIME: 10 TO 15 MINUTES / COOK TIME: 45 TO 55 MINUTES

True to its name, risotto is generally made with short-grain Arborio rice. Its extra starchiness gives this Milanese staple its characteristic creamy texture. I like to use farro in this adaptation because it is high in B vitamins, and the added fiber makes the dish more filling. With a smattering of thyme, a few cups of mushrooms, white wine, and lemon, this asparagus risotto is simple, yet *anything* but boring.

8 to 10 cups unsalted vegetable broth

4 tablespoons extra-virgin olive oil, divided

1 pound asparagus, trimmed and cut in ½-inch pieces

1 medium yellow onion, diced

2 cups chopped mushrooms

Leaves from 3 to 4 sprigs fresh thyme, chopped

2 cups farro

½ cup dry white wine

2 teaspoons kosher salt or sea salt

½ teaspoon freshly ground black pepper

Zest and juice of ½ medium lemon

¼ cup freshly grated Parmesan cheese

1. In a large pot over medium heat, bring the broth to a simmer. Reduce the heat to low, cover the pot, and keep the pot of broth warm for the duration of cooking.

2. In a separate pot or Dutch oven, heat 3 tablespoons of the olive oil over medium heat. Add the asparagus and cook for 4 to 5 minutes, until slightly soft. Remove the asparagus from the pot and set it aside. Add the onion and sauté for 2 to 3 minutes. Stir in the mushrooms and sauté for another 3 to 4 minutes, until the vegetables are soft. Stir in the thyme and farro. Increase heat to medium high. Add the white wine and cook, stirring constantly, until the wine has evaporated.

3. Add one ladle of broth to the pot and cook, stirring constantly, until the liquid is absorbed. Add another ladle of broth, adjusting the heat as needed so the risotto is at a constant simmer. Continue stirring and adding a ladle of broth, allowing the liquid to absorb, until all the broth is used up and the farro is al dente. Season with salt and black pepper throughout the cooking process, then finish by stirring in the lemon

zest and juice, Parmesan cheese, and the asparagus pieces, saving a few for garnish.

4. Divide the risotto among individual serving bowls. Garnish with the remaining asparagus pieces and the remaining tablespoon of olive oil.

5. Store the risotto in an airtight container in the refrigerator for up to 4 days. Reheat it in the microwave on high for 2 to 3 minutes or until heated through.

Variation Tip: Use arborio rice if you're interested in making traditional risotto; this also makes the dish gluten-free. Use any green vegetable in this risotto, such as broccoli or leafy greens, instead of the asparagus (or use all three!).

Cooking Tip: The amount of broth you use when making risotto depends on many factors. I typically heat up more than I think I will need, just in case.

Nutrition Information (per serving): Calories 200; Total fat 8g; Saturated fat 1g; Cholesterol 1mg; Sodium 578mg; Carbs 25g; Fiber 3g; Sugar 7g; Protein 6g

VEGGIE PIZZA WITH CREAMY CAULIFLOWER SAUCE

SERVES 4 / PREP TIME: 20 TO 25 MINUTES / COOK TIME: 15 TO 20 MINUTES

Most people are pizza lovers, and making pizza from scratch is easy and delicious with this recipe! The sauce is made in a blender using cooked cauliflower as the base ingredient, the crust requires zero rising time and is made with whole wheat flour and Greek yogurt, and the toppings are yours to choose. Sprinkle with a little cheese and bake until crispy and bubbly.

For the cauliflower sauce

1 tablespoon extra-virgin olive oil

2 to 3 garlic cloves, minced

2 cups frozen cauliflower florets, thawed

¼ cup unsalted vegetable broth

¼ cup milk

2 tablespoons freshly grated Parmesan cheese

Zest and juice of ½ medium lemon

1 teaspoon kosher salt or sea salt

½ teaspoon freshly ground black pepper

For the crust

1⅓ cups plain Greek yogurt

To make the cauliflower sauce

1. Heat the olive oil in a skillet over medium-low heat. Add the garlic and sauté for 30 to 60 seconds or until fragrant.

2. Transfer the oil and garlic to a blender and add the thawed cauliflower, broth, milk, Parmesan, lemon zest and juice, salt, and black pepper. Purée until smooth. Taste and adjust the seasonings, if necessary.

To make the crust

1. In a bowl, stir together the Greek yogurt, flour, and salt until a dough ball forms. If the dough seems dry, add a few tablespoons of warm water.

2. Transfer the dough to a large cutting board and sprinkle it with a bit more flour. Roll it out into a circle, about ½ inch thick. Transfer the dough to a baking sheet and brush it with the olive oil.

1¾ cups whole wheat all-purpose flour

¼ teaspoon kosher salt or sea salt

1 tablespoon extra-virgin olive oil

For the pizza

2 cups baby spinach

1 cup sliced mushrooms

½ medium green bell pepper, seeded and diced

¼ medium red onion, diced

½ cup sliced olives

1 cup shredded mozzarella cheese

To make the pizza

1. Preheat the oven to 425°F.

2. Spread the cauliflower sauce over the dough. Top with the spinach, mushrooms, bell pepper, red onion, olives, and mozzarella cheese.

3. Bake for 12 to 15 minutes or until the crust is browned and the cheese is bubbly and lightly browned. Remove the pizza from the oven and let it cool slightly, then cut it into 8 slices.

4. Store the pizza in an airtight container in the refrigerator for up to 4 days. Enjoy it cold, or reheat it in the microwave on high for 1 to 3 minutes or until heated through.

Variation Tip: If you are pressed for time, use jarred marinara sauce instead of making the cauliflower sauce. Use any combination of about 3 cups of chopped veggies for the toppings.

Cooking Tip: I use frozen cauliflower florets that have been thawed. You can also steam fresh florets in water on the stove or in the microwave until fork-tender.

Nutrition Information (per serving, 2 slices): Calories 438; Total fat 18g; Saturated fat 5g; Cholesterol 26mg; Sodium 634mg; Carbs 51g; Fiber 9g; Sugar 7g; Protein 24g

MINI VEGGIE POT PIES

SERVES 6 / PREP TIME: 20 TO 25 MINUTES / COOK TIME: 1 HOUR 15 MINUTES

Pot pie is the ultimate comfort food, and it's loaded with brain-healthy veggies, too! I like to make mini pot pies by using individual ramekins, but you can also make this as one big pie in a Dutch oven or casserole dish. The crust is essentially a basic pie crust, but I use whole wheat pastry flour for a boost of nutrition.

For the pot pie filling

2 tablespoons extra-virgin olive oil

1 medium yellow onion, diced

2 medium carrots, peeled and diced

2 medium stalks celery, diced

1 medium Yukon Gold or red potato, diced (skin-on)

1 cup green or red lentils

½ cup dry white wine

4 to 5 cups unsalted vegetable broth

1 cup frozen peas

2 teaspoons Worcestershire sauce

Leaves from 2 sprigs fresh thyme, chopped

Leaves from 1 sprig fresh rosemary, chopped

1¾ teaspoons kosher salt or sea salt

To make the pot pie filling

1. Heat the olive oil in a Dutch oven or stockpot over medium heat. Add the onion, carrots, and celery and sauté for 4 to 5 minutes or until the vegetables are soft. Add the potato, lentils, and white wine and simmer, stirring constantly, until the wine has been absorbed. Add the broth, bring it to a simmer, and cook for 25 to 30 minutes or until the potatoes and lentils are tender.

2. Stir in the peas, Worcestershire sauce, thyme, rosemary, salt, and black pepper. Cook for an additional 2 to 3 minutes or until the peas are hot. Taste and adjust the seasonings, if necessary.

3. In a small bowl, whisk together the milk and cornstarch; pour this mixture into the pot. Cook for another 1 to 2 minutes or until the mixture is thickened.

4. Coat 8 ramekins with cooking spray. Transfer the pot pie filling to the ramekins.

5. Preheat the oven to 375°F.

To make the crust

1. In a large mixing bowl, stir together the flour and salt. Add the cubed butter and 4 tablespoons of

½ teaspoon freshly ground black pepper

¼ cup milk

1 tablespoon cornstarch

Nonstick cooking spray

For the crust

1 ¼ cups whole wheat pastry flour

½ teaspoon kosher salt or sea salt

4 tablespoons cold unsalted butter, cubed

4 to 5 tablespoons ice water

1 large egg, beaten

the ice water, and use a fork or pastry cutter to cut the butter cubes into the flour until small, pea-size granules form. Add the remaining tablespoon of ice water if needed to help the dough come together.

2. Transfer the dough to a cutting board and sprinkle with a bit more flour. Work the dough into a ball, then roll it out into a circle, about ¼ inch thick. Use a coffee cup to cut out six rounds.

To make the pot pies

1. Place a dough round on top of each ramekin. Brush the dough with the beaten egg. Bake for 25 to 30 minutes or until the topping is lightly browned and crispy.

2. Refrigerate the pot pies in the ramekins, covered, for up to 4 days. Reheat them in a 375°F oven for 15 to 20 minutes, or microwave for 3 to 4 minutes, until heated through.

Variation Tip: Use coconut oil instead of butter, if desired. For a meat version, use chicken or turkey in place of or in addition to the lentils.

Cooking Tip: You can use a food processor to make the crust. Simply pulse the flour, salt, and butter, and drizzle in the ice water until pea-size granules form.

Nutrition Information (per serving): Calories 343; Total fat 14g; Saturated fat 6g; Cholesterol 31mg; Sodium 587mg; Carbs 43g; Fiber 8g; Sugar 7g; Protein 10g

RAINBOW VEGGIE SPRING ROLLS

SERVES 5 / PREP TIME: 20 TO 30 MINUTES

Spring rolls can seem intimidating to make, but they're actually quite simple and fun! Once the rice papers have soaked in water for a minute or two, you add raw veggies to the center of each one, roll them up like burritos, and serve with a simple dipping sauce. They make a great meal or snack.

For the spring rolls

10 (8-inch) spring roll wrappers or rice papers

2 medium ripe avocados, pitted and sliced

1 large English cucumber, julienned

1 medium red bell pepper, seeded and cut into strips

1 cup julienned carrots

1 cup shredded purple cabbage

½ small jalapeño, seeded and thinly sliced (optional)

1 cup fresh cilantro leaves

Juice of 2 medium limes

For the dipping sauce

2 tablespoons low-sodium soy sauce

2 teaspoons sesame oil

1 teaspoon honey

¼ teaspoon crushed red pepper flakes

To make the spring rolls

1. Pour an inch or so of room temperature water into a 9-inch round pan or pie plate. Working one at a time, soak the spring roll wrappers in the water for 45 to 60 seconds, until they feel soft and pliable. Transfer the soaked wrappers to a flat surface and pat them dry.

2. In the center of each wrapper, stack an avocado slice, about ¼ cup vegetables, and a few cilantro leaves; top with a squeeze of lime juice. Fold the ends of each wrapper over the vegetables, then roll it up like a burrito.

3. Repeat steps 1 and 2 until all the fillings are used up.

To make the dipping sauce

1. In a small bowl, whisk together the soy sauce, sesame oil, honey, and crushed red pepper flakes; serve with the spring rolls.

2. Store the spring rolls in an airtight container in the refrigerator for up to 3 days. Store the dipping sauce in a separate container in the refrigerator for up to 5 days.

Variation Tip: Add cooked, peeled, and deveined shrimp for a seafood version. Try julienned radishes instead of red bell pepper.

Cooking Tip: To julienne means to thinly slice vegetables into matchsticks.

Nutrition Information (per serving, 2 rolls): Calories 302; Total fat 11g; Saturated fat 2g; Cholesterol 0mg; Sodium 362mg; Carbs 52g; Fiber 8g; Sugar 7g; Protein 3g

THAI-STYLE CAULIFLOWER-WALNUT LETTUCE CUPS

SERVES 6 / PREP TIME: 10 TO 15 MINUTES / COOK TIME: 15 TO 20 MINUTES

The ginger, lime zest and juice, and cilantro give this cauliflower-walnut filling a deliciously unique flavor. The honey provides a touch of sweetness and balances the tart ingredients, and the jalapeño brings a bit of heat. Serving this in Bibb lettuce cups gives it an additional burst of nutrition and freshness.

4 to 5 cups cauliflower florets

1½ cups chopped unsalted walnuts

3 tablespoons avocado oil or canola oil

½ medium yellow onion, finely diced

½ small jalapeño, seeded and minced

3 to 4 garlic cloves, minced

3-inch piece fresh ginger, peeled and minced

3½ tablespoons low-sodium soy sauce

Zest and juice of 1 medium lime

1 tablespoon honey

1 teaspoon sesame oil

½ teaspoon kosher salt or sea salt

1. Place the cauliflower florets in the bowl of a food processor and pulse until they are chopped into pea-size pieces.

2. Heat a large skillet over medium-low heat. Add the chopped walnuts and toast for 1 to 3 minutes or until fragrant, shaking the pan to keep the walnuts from burning. Transfer to a bowl and set aside.

3. In the same skillet, heat the oil over medium heat. Add the cauliflower pieces, onion, and jalapeño and sauté for 5 to 6 minutes or until the vegetables are soft. Stir in the garlic and ginger and sauté for an additional 1 to 2 minutes or until the garlic is fragrant.

4. Add the soy sauce, lime zest and juice, honey, and sesame oil and increase the heat to medium high. Simmer for 3 to 4 minutes, stirring frequently, until thickened. Stir in the toasted walnuts, salt, and cilantro.

5. Scoop the mixture into the lettuce leaves and top with the green onions. Serve immediately.

½ cup fresh cilantro leaves, chopped

Large leaves from 2 heads Bibb lettuce (about 12 leaves)

3 green onions, thinly sliced

6. Store the filling in an airtight container in the refrigerator for up to 4 days. Enjoy it cold, or reheat it in the microwave for 1 to 2 minutes, until heated through. Refrigerate the lettuce leaves in a sealed plastic bag with a paper towel to absorb moisture.

Variation Tip: Use low-sodium tamari instead of soy sauce for a gluten-free version. Add a dash of vegan fish sauce (or regular fish sauce) for extra flavor. Serve the cauliflower-walnut mixture on top of rice instead of in lettuce cups.

Cooking Tip: You can skip step 1 of the instructions by using pre-riced cauliflower; it can be found in bags in the produce section or freezer aisle of your grocery store.

Nutrition Information (per serving, 2 wraps): Calories 339; Total fat 27g; Saturated fat 3g; Cholesterol 0mg; Sodium 650mg; Carbs 18g; Fiber 6g; Sugar 8g; Protein 10g

APPLE AND WILD RICE–STUFFED ACORN SQUASH

SERVES 4 / PREP TIME: 10 TO 15 MINUTES / COOK TIME: 1 HOUR

Acorn squash halves make the perfect cups for delicious stuffing. This one calls for wild rice, apples, dried cranberries, and pecans. Once the squash halves are baked, drizzle them with a bit of maple syrup for a beautiful fall dinner.

Nonstick cooking spray

2 medium acorn squash, halved and seeded

3 tablespoons extra-virgin olive oil

½ medium yellow onion, diced

1 medium Granny Smith apple, cored and diced (skin-on)

2 to 3 garlic cloves, minced

1 cup cooked wild rice

1½ tablespoons chopped fresh sage

1½ teaspoons kosher salt or sea salt, divided

½ teaspoon freshly ground black pepper

¼ to ½ cup unsalted vegetable broth

½ cup unsweetened dried cranberries

¼ cup chopped unsalted pecans

1. Preheat the oven to 400°F. Grease a baking dish with cooking spray.

2. Lay the acorn squash halves cut-side down in the prepared baking dish. Roast for 30 to 40 minutes or until fork tender.

3. Meanwhile, heat the olive oil in a Dutch oven or stockpot over medium heat. Add the onion and sauté for 2 to 3 minutes, then add the apple and sauté for an additional 2 to 3 minutes, until slightly soft. Stir in the garlic, wild rice, sage, 1¼ teaspoons of the salt, and the black pepper. Add the broth and bring it to a simmer, then cook, stirring occasionally, for 5 to 10 minutes or until the broth is absorbed.

4. Stir the cranberries and pecans into the wild rice mixture. Taste and adjust the seasonings, if necessary.

5. When the squash is done roasting, remove it from the oven and flip the halves so the cut sides are facing up. Drizzle the wells of the squash with the maple syrup and sprinkle with the cinnamon and remaining ¼ teaspoon of salt. Spoon the wild rice mixture into the wells of the squash.

2 tablespoons pure maple
syrup

1 teaspoon ground cinnamon

6. Store the stuffed squash in an airtight container in the refrigerator for up to 4 days. Reheat them in the microwave for 2 to 3 minutes or until heated through.

Variation Tip: Use walnuts instead of pecans. Use fresh cranberries when they are in season: Add ½ cup of them to the pan with the apples, add an extra ¼ cup of broth, and simmer with the wild rice until the cranberries burst.

Cooking Tip: Cook the wild rice ahead of time: Bring ¾ cup of water to a simmer and add ¼ cup of wild rice. Cover and cook over medium-low heat for 45 to 60 minutes, stirring occasionally. Drain any excess water.

Nutrition Information (per serving): Calories 345; Total fat 16g; Saturated fat 2g; Cholesterol 0mg; Sodium 444mg; Carbs 53g; Fiber 8g; Sugar 14g; Protein 4g

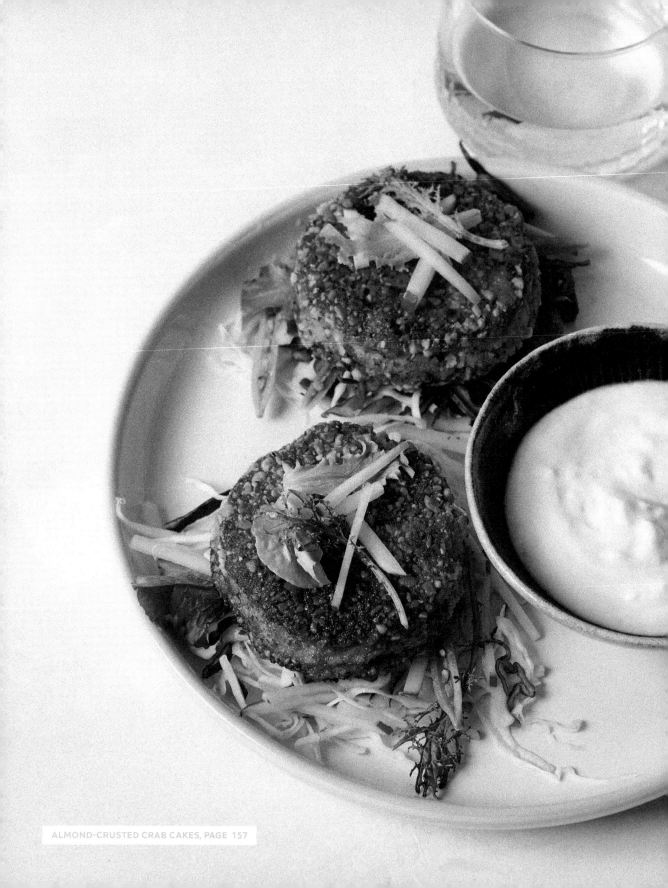

ALMOND-CRUSTED CRAB CAKES, PAGE 157

CHAPTER SEVEN

Seafood Mains

SHRIMP AND ROASTED RED PEPPER GRITS

SERVES 6 / PREP TIME: 10 TO 15 MINUTES / COOK TIME: 20 TO 30 MINUTES

Grits are a type of creamy porridge made with coarsely ground cornmeal. They are often served with sautéed shrimp for a Southern-style main dish, but in this recipe I've added a bunch of Swiss chard for a pop of beautiful color and a boost of nutrition.

For the grits

2 cups unsalted vegetable broth or chicken stock

2½ cups milk

1 cup cornmeal

½ teaspoon kosher salt or sea salt

½ teaspoon freshly ground black pepper

2 tablespoons unsalted butter

¼ cup chopped roasted red peppers

To make the grits

1. Bring the broth and milk to a simmer in a large saucepan over medium heat. Whisk in the cornmeal, salt, and black pepper. Simmer, stirring frequently, for about 15 minutes, until the mixture is soft and thickened.

2. Remove the pan from the heat, and stir in the butter and roasted red peppers.

To cook the shrimp

1. In a large skillet, heat the olive oil over medium heat. Add the shrimp and sprinkle with ¼ teaspoon salt; cook for 2 minutes per side, until the shrimp are slightly crispy on the edges. Remove the shrimp and place them on a plate.

2. Add the Swiss chard and garlic to the skillet and sauté for 3 to 4 minutes or until the chard is wilted. Add the shrimp back to the skillet and stir in the lemon zest and juice, remaining ¼ teaspoon salt, and black pepper.

For the shrimp

2 tablespoons extra-virgin olive oil

1¼ pounds large raw shrimp, peeled and deveined, tails removed

½ teaspoon kosher salt or sea salt, divided

1 bunch Swiss chard, stemmed and chopped

3 to 4 garlic cloves, minced

Zest and juice of ½ medium lemon

¼ teaspoon freshly ground black pepper

3. Spoon the grits into bowls and top with the shrimp and chard mixture.

4. Store the shrimp and grits in an airtight container in the refrigerator for up to 4 days. Reheat by microwaving on high for 1 to 3 minutes or until heated through.

Variation Tip: Try using instant polenta instead of cornmeal. Try spinach, kale, mustard greens, or turnips greens instead of Swiss chard.

Cooking Tip: You can use yellow or white cornmeal to make grits; a coarse cut is best.

Nutrition Information (per serving): Calories 288; Total fat 10g; Saturated fat 6g; Cholesterol 196mg; Sodium 668mg; Carbs 25g; Fiber 1g; Sugar 8g; Protein 25g

SHRIMP-PEANUT PAD THAI

SERVES 8 / PREP TIME: 20 TO 25 MINUTES / COOK TIME: 15 TO 20 MINUTES

The peanut sauce in this pad thai is out-of-this-world. In this recipe, it's tossed with rice noodles, shrimp, and scrambled eggs. Your family won't believe it didn't come from a Thai restaurant!

For the peanut sauce

¼ cup natural peanut butter

2 tablespoons brown sugar

2 tablespoons soy sauce

Zest and juice of
1 medium lime

½ tablespoon fish sauce

2 teaspoons sesame oil

2-inch piece fresh ginger,
peeled and minced

For the pad thai

8 ounces brown rice noodles

Nonstick cooking spray

2 large eggs, beaten

½ teaspoon kosher salt or sea
salt, divided

2 tablespoons avocado oil or
canola oil

1½ pounds large raw shrimp,
peeled and deveined, tails
removed

2 medium shallots, thinly
sliced

3 to 4 garlic cloves, minced

3 to 4 green onions, thinly
sliced

½ cup unsalted peanuts,
crushed

To make the peanut sauce

In a small bowl, whisk together the peanut butter, brown sugar, soy sauce, lime zest and juice, fish sauce, sesame oil, ginger, and a splash of hot water. Set aside.

To make the pad thai

1. Place the noodles in a large bowl, and cover them with boiling water. Soak for 5 to 6 minutes, then drain.

2. Heat a large skillet over medium-low heat, and coat it with cooking spray. Add the beaten eggs, season with ¼ teaspoon salt, and cook for 3 to 4 minutes, using a spatula to constantly scramble them until they are fluffy and cooked through. Transfer the eggs to a plate.

3. In the same skillet, heat the oil over medium heat. Add the shrimp and cook for 2 minutes per side, until slightly crispy on the edges. Stir in the shallots and garlic and sprinkle with the remaining ¼ teaspoon salt; cook for 1 to 3 minutes or until the garlic is fragrant. Stir in the peanut sauce and bring it to a simmer. Add the noodles and scrambled eggs, then immediately toss continuously, using tongs, until everything is well incorporated.

4. Scoop the pad thai into bowls, and top with the green onions and peanuts.

5. Store the pad thai in an airtight container in the refrigerator for up to 4 days. Enjoy it cold, or reheat it by microwaving on high for 1 to 3 minutes, until heated through.

Variation Tip: If you can't find rice noodles, use spaghetti or linguine. Try chicken instead of shrimp.

Cooking Tip: For an extra nutty flavor, toast the peanuts in a hot, dry skillet for 30 to 60 seconds before adding them to the recipe.

Make It a Meal: Serve with stir-fried vegetables.

Nutrition Information (per serving): Calories 396; Total fat 16g; Saturated fat 2g; Cholesterol 221mg; Sodium 516mg; Carbs 32g; Fiber 2g; Sugar 5g; Protein 31g

GLUTEN-FREE

LEMONY GARLIC SHRIMP SCAMPI

SERVES 6 / PREP TIME: 20 TO 25 MINUTES / COOK TIME: 15 TO 20 MINUTES

Shrimp scampi can be served on its own, but when it's paired with spaghetti it becomes more filling and satisfying. You can add a few cups of chopped dark leafy greens, or you can serve it as-is with a side salad or grilled, roasted, or sautéed vegetables to make it a complete meal.

8 ounces whole-grain spaghetti

3 tablespoons extra-virgin olive oil, divided

2 pounds large raw shrimp, peeled and deveined, tails removed

1 teaspoon kosher salt or sea salt, divided

4 to 5 garlic cloves, minced

1 cup dry white wine

Zest and juice of ½ medium lemon

1 tablespoon unsalted butter

¼ teaspoon crushed red pepper flakes

¼ cup fresh flat-leaf Italian parsley leaves, chopped

1. Bring a large pot of water to a boil. Cook the pasta according to the package directions.

2. Reserve ½ cup of the pasta water, then drain the pasta. Set the pasta aside.

3. In a large skillet, heat 1 tablespoon of the olive oil over medium heat. Add the shrimp and sprinkle with ½ teaspoon of the salt. Cook the shrimp for 2 minutes per side, until slightly crispy on the edges. Remove the shrimp and place them on a plate. Set aside.

4. Add the garlic to the skillet and sauté for 1 to 3 minutes. Add the reserved pasta water, white wine, and lemon zest and juice; and simmer until the liquid is reduced, about 2 to 3 minutes.

5. Reduce the heat and stir in the cooked shrimp, butter, remaining ½ teaspoon of salt, red pepper flakes, and chopped parsley. Cook for an additional 2 to 3 minutes or until the shrimp is fully cooked. Add the pasta and the remaining 2 tablespoons of olive oil; toss to coat. Serve immediately.

6. Store the shrimp scampi in an airtight container in the refrigerator for up to 4 days. Reheat it by microwaving on high for 1 to 3 minutes, until heated through.

Variation Tip: Try scallops instead of shrimp. Try protein-enriched pasta for a meal that'll keep you full for hours.

Cooking Tip: It's optional, but adding salt to the pasta water instills flavor in the pasta and keeps it from sticking together.

Nutrition Information (per serving): Calories 405; Total fat 12g; Saturated fat 6g; Cholesterol 298mg; Sodium 393mg; Carbs 30g; Fiber 4g; Sugar 2g; Protein 36g

CITRUS-MARINATED COCONUT SHRIMP

SERVES 6 / PREP TIME: 40 TO 45 MINUTES / COOK TIME: 10 TO 15 MINUTES

Despite the name, marinating the shrimp in orange and lime juice is optional in this dish, but I highly suggest it! It takes crispy coconut shrimp from really good—to really, *really* great. The coconut batter gets crispy in the oven, so you don't even miss the fact that it's not deep-fried. Plus, the orange preserves and sweet chili sauce combination to dip them in is out-of-this-world.

For the marinade
Zest and juice of 2 medium oranges

Zest and juice of 6 medium limes

3 tablespoons extra-virgin olive oil

1 to 2 garlic cloves, minced

½ teaspoon kosher salt or sea salt

¼ teaspoon freshly ground black pepper

For the shrimp
1½ pounds large raw shrimp, peeled and deveined, tails removed

Nonstick cooking spray

¾ cup all-purpose flour

2 large eggs, beaten

1 cup panko breadcrumbs

5 tablespoons unsweetened shredded coconut

To make the marinade
In a large glass bowl, whisk together the orange zest and juice, lime zest and juice, olive oil, garlic, salt, and black pepper.

To make the shrimp
1. Add the shrimp to the marinade and toss to coat.

2. Cover the bowl and refrigerate for 30 minutes. Remove the shrimp from the bowl and place them on a paper towel–lined plate. Pat them dry. Discard the marinade.

3. Preheat the oven to 400°F. Place a wire rack inside a baking sheet, and coat it with cooking spray.

4. Set up 3 bowls: one with the flour, one with the beaten egg, and one with the panko and shredded coconut. Divide the salt and black pepper among the bowls, and stir each to combine.

5. Working one at a time, dip the shrimp into the flour, then the egg, and then the panko-coconut mixture, and place them on the prepared wire rack. Coat each piece of shrimp with cooking spray. Bake for 10 to 15 minutes or until the shrimp are firm.

½ teaspoon kosher or
sea salt

¼ teaspoon ground black
pepper

For the dipping sauce

3 tablespoons orange
preserves

2 tablespoons sweet chili
sauce

To make the dipping sauce

1. In a small bowl, whisk together the orange preserves and chili sauce. Serve the coconut shrimp with the dipping sauce.

2. Store the coconut shrimp in an airtight container in the refrigerator for up to 4 days. Reheat by toasting the shrimp under the broiler until crispy. Store the dipping sauce in an airtight container in the refrigerator for up to 7 days.

Variation Tip: Use gluten-free all-purpose flour and panko breadcrumbs for a gluten-free version.

Cooking Tip: Skip the marinating step if you're in a rush.

Make It a Meal: Serve with a side of roasted, grilled, or steamed vegetables or a green salad.

Nutrition Information (per serving): Calories 328; Total fat 10g; Saturated fat 5g; Cholesterol 282mg; Sodium 558mg; Carbs 29g; Fiber 2g; Sugar 11g; Protein 29g

TUNA BURGERS WITH SCALLION AIOLI

MAKES 4 BURGERS / PREP TIME: 10 TO 15 MINUTES / COOK TIME: 8 TO 10 MINUTES

These tuna burgers have the most amazing mixture of Asian-inspired flavors. You can use fresh tuna or swap in canned or pouched tuna for a quick and easy burger. Either way, you'll love them!

For the burgers

1 pound fresh ahi tuna

3 green onions, thinly sliced

2-inch piece fresh ginger, peeled and minced

3 to 4 garlic cloves, minced

2 tablespoons low-sodium soy sauce

1½ teaspoons sesame oil

1 teaspoon sriracha sauce

½ teaspoon kosher salt or sea salt

½ teaspoon freshly ground black pepper

3 tablespoons avocado oil or canola oil

For the aioli

¼ cup mayonnaise

Zest and juice of ½ medium lime

2 green onions, thinly sliced

To make the burgers

1. Place the tuna in a food processor and pulse until it is ground. Transfer the tuna to a bowl. To the bowl, add the green onions, ginger, garlic, soy sauce, sesame oil, sriracha, salt, and black pepper; mix until thoroughly combined. Form the mixture into four patties.

2. In a large skillet, heat the oil over medium heat. Add the tuna patties and cook for 3 to 4 minutes per side or until their internal temperature reaches 145°F.

To make the aioli

1. In a small bowl, stir together the mayonnaise, lime zest and juice, and green onions.

2. Serve the tuna burgers on their own topped with aioli, or serve them in lettuce cups or on whole-grain buns.

3. Store the burgers in an airtight container in the refrigerator for up to 4 days. Reheat them by microwaving on high for 1 to 3 minutes, until heated through. Store the aioli in a separate airtight container for up to 4 days.

Variation Tip: Try salmon instead of tuna.

Cooking Tip: To achieve a crispy crust on the tuna burger, let the pan get very hot before adding the burgers.

Make It a Meal: Serve with a side of roasted, grilled, or steamed vegetables or a green salad.

Nutrition Information (per serving, 1 burger): Calories 344; Total fat 23g; Saturated fat 3g; Cholesterol 50mg; Sodium 654mg; Carbs 5g; Fiber 1g; Sugar 1g; Protein 29g

TUNA AND AVOCADO EGG SALAD

SERVES 6 / PREP TIME: 10 TO 15 MINUTES / COOK TIME: 17 TO 18 MINUTES

The hard-boiled eggs can be prepped in advance, so this salad comes together in just minutes. Because it's high in protein and packed with brain- and heart-healthy monounsaturated fats, it will keep you full for hours. The lemon juice and parsley give the salad fresh flavors, while the avocado and mayonnaise make it creamy and rich.

8 large eggs

2 medium ripe avocados, halved, pitted, and peeled

12 ounces canned or pouched albacore tuna, drained

Zest and juice of ½ medium lemon

1 tablespoon mayonnaise

¼ cup fresh flat-leaf Italian parsley leaves, chopped

¼ teaspoon kosher salt or sea salt

¼ teaspoon freshly ground black pepper

1. Place the eggs in a saucepan and cover them with cold water. Bring to a boil over medium-high heat, shut off the heat, and cover the pan with a fitted lid. Set a timer for 17 minutes. When the timer goes off, drain the hot water and pour ice water over the eggs until they are cool enough to handle. Peel the eggs and cut them into bite-size pieces.

2. In a bowl, mash the avocados. Add the eggs to the bowl, along with the tuna, lemon zest and juice, mayonnaise, parsley, salt, and black pepper; stir to combine.

3. Store the salad in an airtight container in the refrigerator for up to 4 days.

Variation Tip: Try canned or pouched salmon or crab. Skip the boiled egg to make tuna avocado salad, or skip the tuna to make avocado egg salad.

Cooking Tip: Use eggs that are at least a week old, as they're easier to peel.

Nutrition Information (per serving): Calories 261; Total fat 15g; Saturated fat 3g; Cholesterol 269mg; Sodium 341mg; Carbs 5g; Fiber 3g; Sugar 1g; Protein 25g

MINI DILL-SALMON CAKES

MAKES 12 CAKES / PREP TIME: 10 TO 15 MINUTES / COOK TIME: 15 TO 20 MINUTES

Depending on their size, salmon cakes can be served as appetizers or main courses. You can use dried or fresh dill: If you use dried, use only 1 tablespoon, as it's much more potent than fresh.

20 ounces canned or pouched salmon, drained

½ cup panko breadcrumbs

2 large eggs

3 tablespoons extra-virgin olive oil, divided

2 tablespoons Dijon mustard

2 tablespoons chopped fresh dill

Zest and juice of ½ medium lemon

2 teaspoons dried oregano

¾ teaspoon kosher salt or sea salt

½ teaspoon freshly ground black pepper

¼ teaspoon crushed red pepper flakes

1. Place the salmon, panko, eggs, 1 tablespoon of the olive oil, Dijon mustard, dill, lemon zest and juice, oregano, salt, black pepper, and crushed red pepper flakes in a bowl; stir to combine.

2. Form the mixture into 12 (2-inch) patties.

3. Heat the remaining 2 tablespoons of olive oil in a large skillet over medium heat. Working in two batches, cook the patties for 3 to 4 minutes per side, until the exterior is browned and crispy and the patties are firm.

4. Store the salmon cakes in an airtight container in the refrigerator for up to 2 days. Reheat them by microwaving on high for 1 to 3 minutes, until heated through.

Variation Tip: Use gluten-free breadcrumbs for a gluten-free version. Serve on buns or in lettuce cups with dollops of plain Greek yogurt.

Cooking Tip: Bake them instead—simply place them on a greased baking sheet and cook at 375°F until firm, about 10 to 12 minutes.

Nutrition Information (per serving, 2 cakes): Calories 214; Total fat 11g; Saturated fat 2g; Cholesterol 95mg; Sodium 570mg; Carbs 5g; Fiber 0g; Sugar 1g; Protein 24g

HONEY MUSTARD GRILLED SALMON

SERVES 4 / PREP TIME: 5 TO 10 MINUTES / COOK TIME: 15 TO 20 MINUTES

Talk about a quick and easy way to get in your omega-3s! This salmon recipe has only a few staple ingredients but phenomenal flavor. The versatile, two-ingredient honey-Dijon sauce tastes delicious on the salmon as well as on chicken and pork dishes.

3 tablespoons honey

3 tablespoons Dijon mustard

1 pound fresh salmon fillets, skin on

1 tablespoon avocado oil or canola oil

½ teaspoon kosher salt or sea salt

¼ teaspoon freshly ground black pepper

1. Preheat a grill to medium heat.

2. In a small bowl, whisk together the honey and Dijon.

3. Brush the salmon with the oil and season it on both sides with salt and black pepper. Place the salmon flesh-side down on the grill and cook for 4 to 6 minutes. Flip the fillets, then brush the tops with the honey mustard mixture. Cook for another 4 to 6 minutes or until the salmon flakes easily with a fork. Serve immediately.

4. Store the salmon in an airtight container in the refrigerator for up to 2 days. Reheat it by microwaving on high for 1 to 3 minutes until heated through.

Variation Tip: Try pure maple syrup instead of honey. Rather than grilling, broil the salmon for 8 to 12 minutes.

Cooking Tip: Use a fork to test the doneness of the salmon. Press the thickest part of the salmon with the back of a fork; if it starts to fall apart, it's done. If it springs back, it's not quite done.

Make It a Meal: Serve with a green salad or a side of roasted, grilled, or steamed vegetables.

Nutrition Information (per serving): Calories 239; Total fat 11g; Saturated fat 1g; Cholesterol 50mg; Sodium 191mg; Carbs 13g; Fiber 0g; Sugar 13g; Protein 22g

SESAME-GINGER GLAZED SALMON

SERVES 6 / PREP TIME: 30 TO 45 MINUTES / COOK TIME: 15 TO 20 MINUTES

This soy and honey sauce is reminiscent of teriyaki and gives the salmon a rich, sweet, and tangy flavor that can't be beat. Marinating imparts more flavor to the salmon, but if you're in a hurry, you can skip that step and simply brush the salmon with the sauce as it cooks.

For the marinade

3 tablespoons low-sodium soy sauce

2 tablespoons honey

1 tablespoon rice wine vinegar

1½ teaspoons sesame oil

2 to 3 garlic cloves, minced

2-inch piece fresh ginger, peeled and minced

For the salmon

1½ pounds fresh salmon fillets, skin on

Nonstick cooking spray

2 tablespoons unsalted vegetable broth

1 tablespoon cornstarch

3 tablespoons sesame seeds

2 green onions, thinly sliced

To make the marinade

Place the soy sauce, honey, rice wine vinegar, sesame oil, garlic, and ginger in a gallon-size zip-top bag; seal the bag and shake it around to mix. Add the salmon fillets, seal the bag, and refrigerate for 30 minutes.

To make the salmon

1. Preheat the broiler. Coat a baking sheet with cooking spray. Use tongs to transfer the marinated salmon fillets to the baking sheet, skin-sides down. Broil for 8 to 10 minutes or until the salmon flakes easily with a fork.

2. Meanwhile, pour the marinade into a saucepan and bring it to a simmer over medium heat. In a small bowl, whisk together the broth and cornstarch until combined. Pour the cornstarch slurry into the saucepan, bring the mixture to a simmer, and whisk until thickened.

3. Pour the sauce over the salmon fillets and garnish with the sesame seeds and green onions. Serve immediately.

4. Store the salmon in an airtight container in the refrigerator for up to 2 days. Reheat it by microwaving on high for 1 to 3 minutes, until heated through.

Variation Tip: Try this sauce on sautéed shrimp.

Cooking Tip: Store fresh ginger in a sealable plastic bag in the freezer for up to 3 months.

Make It a Meal: Serve with a green salad or a side of roasted, grilled, or steamed vegetables.

Nutrition Information (per serving): Calories 228; Total fat 10g; Saturated fat 1g; Cholesterol 50mg; Sodium 392mg; Carbs 9g; Fiber 1g; Sugar 6g; Protein 23g

SALMON SALAD SANDWICHES

SERVES 6 / PREP TIME: 10 TO 15 MINUTES

Canned salmon and tuna are lifesavers when it comes to whipping up a healthy meal in no time! I recommend keeping some in your pantry to use in salads, casseroles, and pasta dishes when you're in a pinch. This can help you reach the recommended number of servings of omega-3-rich fish per week.

4 tablespoons mayonnaise

2 tablespoons plain yogurt (not Greek)

1 tablespoon Dijon mustard

Zest and juice of ¼ medium lemon

1 tablespoon chopped fresh dill

¼ teaspoon kosher salt or sea salt

¼ teaspoon freshly ground black pepper

⅛ teaspoon cayenne pepper

20 ounces canned or pouched salmon, drained

3 medium stalks celery, diced

2 green onions, thinly sliced

12 Bibb lettuce leaves or 12 slices whole-grain bread

1. In a glass bowl, whisk together the mayonnaise, yogurt, Dijon, lemon zest and juice, dill, salt, black pepper, and cayenne. Fold in the salmon, celery, and green onions. Taste and adjust the seasonings, if necessary.

2. Serve the salmon salad inside Bibb lettuce cups or on slices of whole-grain bread.

3. Store the salmon salad in an airtight container in the refrigerator for up to 3 days.

Variation Tip: Try canned or pouched tuna instead of salmon. Add a tablespoon or two of capers for a briny flavor.

Cooking Tip: For a chilled, more flavorful salad, combine the ingredients, then cover and refrigerate for at least 30 minutes before serving.

Nutrition Information (per serving, 2 lettuce cups): Calories 190; Total fat 9g; Saturated fat 1g; Cholesterol 38mg; Sodium 530mg; Carbs 3g; Fiber 2g; Sugar 2g; Protein 23g

ALMOND-CRUSTED CRAB CAKES

SERVES 8 / PREP TIME: 10 TO 15 MINUTES / COOK TIME: 15 TO 20 MINUTES

Crab cakes are packed with protein and can be served on a bun or lettuce cup, on top of slaws or salads, or with Greek yogurt for dipping. The trick to making perfect crab cakes is to not overcook them. They only need to cook for 3 to 4 minutes per side.

½ **cup sliced unsalted almonds**

¾ teaspoon kosher salt or sea salt, divided

12 ounces lump crab meat or imitation crab

2 large eggs

½ cup panko breadcrumbs

¼ cup fresh flat-leaf Italian parsley leaves

Zest and juice of ½ medium lemon

1 tablespoon Dijon mustard

1½ teaspoons dried oregano

¼ teaspoon freshly ground black pepper

2 tablespoons extra-virgin olive oil

1. Place the almonds and ¼ teaspoon of the salt in the bowl of a food processor. Pulse until they resemble crumbs; transfer to a shallow dish.

2. Place the crab meat, eggs, breadcrumbs, parsley, lemon zest and juice, Dijon mustard, oregano, remaining ½ teaspoon salt, and black pepper in the food processor. Pulse until a paste forms.

3. Form the crab mixture into eight patties, then dredge them in the almond crumbs so all sides are covered.

4. Heat the olive oil in a large skillet over medium heat. Working in two batches, cook the patties for 3 to 4 minutes per side, until the exterior is browned and crispy and the patties are firm.

5. Store the crab cakes in an airtight container in the refrigerator for up to 2 days. Reheat them by toasting under the broiler until hot.

Cooking Tip: You can also bake the crab cakes at 375°F for 8 to 12 minutes.

Make It a Meal: Serve with Greek-Style Orzo (page 101).

Nutrition Information (per serving, 1 crab cake): Calories 251; Total fat 15g; Saturated fat 2g; Cholesterol 191mg; Sodium 594mg; Carbs 7g; Fiber 2g; Sugar 1g; Protein 23g

WHITE FISH NUGGETS

SERVES 6 / PREP TIME: 15 TO 20 MINUTES / COOK TIME: 10 TO 15 MINUTES

Every summer, we drive through northern Michigan on our way to a campsite, and we stop at a small restaurant that serves white fish nuggets. They're fresh out of Lake Michigan and taste juicy and delicious. This is my healthier take on these nuggets, and even though they're baked instead of fried, they're still golden brown and crispy.

For the fish nuggets
Nonstick cooking spray

¾ cup all-purpose flour

2 large eggs, beaten

2 tablespoons Dijon mustard

1¼ cups panko breadcrumbs

1 teaspoon kosher salt or sea salt, divided

¾ teaspoon freshly ground black pepper, divided

1½ **pounds fresh white fish fillets, skin removed, cubed**

For the tartar sauce
2 tablespoons mayonnaise

2 tablespoons plain yogurt (not Greek)

2 tablespoons dill pickle relish

½ tablespoon Dijon mustard

¼ teaspoon freshly ground black pepper

To make the fish nuggets

1. Preheat the oven to 400°F. Place a wire rack inside a baking sheet, and coat it with cooking spray.

2. Set up three bowls: one with the flour, one with the beaten egg and Dijon, and one with the panko. Divide the salt and black pepper among the bowls, and stir each to combine.

3. Working one at a time, dip the fish cubes into the flour, then the egg, and then the panko, and place them on the prepared wire rack. Coat each cube with cooking spray. Bake for 10 to 15 minutes or until the fish is firm.

To make the tartar sauce

1. In a small bowl, whisk together the mayonnaise, yogurt, relish, Dijon, and black pepper. Serve the fish nuggets with the tartar sauce.

2. Store the fish nuggets in an airtight container in the refrigerator for up to 4 days. Reheat by toasting them in the broiler until crispy. Store the tartar sauce in a separate airtight container in the refrigerator for up to 4 days.

Variation Tip: Use chicken or turkey instead of fish.

Cooking Tip: Any white fish will work for this recipe. Try cod, haddock, halibut, tilapia, or catfish. If making the nuggets with catfish, swap in cornmeal for the panko.

Make It a Meal: Serve with Spinach, Strawberry, and Fennel Salad (page 85).

Nutrition Information (per serving): Calories 232; Total fat 6g; Saturated fat 1g; Cholesterol 113mg; Sodium 326mg; Carbs 17g; Fiber 1g; Sugar 1g; Protein 25g

FISH TACOS WITH CABBAGE SLAW

SERVES 6 / PREP TIME: 15 TO 20 MINUTES / COOK TIME: 10 TO 15 MINUTES

Fish tacos are my favorite California street food, and you can easily make them at home. I rub the fish with a spice mixture and then pan-fry them until tender and flaky, but you can also bread and bake the fish using the same method I used to make the White Fish Nuggets (page 158). Finish off the tacos with heaping spoonfuls of citrus slaw and some creamy avocado slices.

For the slaw

Zest and juice of 2 medium limes

3 tablespoons avocado oil or canola oil

1 tablespoon honey

½ teaspoon kosher salt or sea salt

3 cups shredded green, red, or Napa cabbage or coleslaw mix

For the fish

1½ tablespoons chili powder

1 teaspoon ground cumin

1 teaspoon kosher salt or sea salt

½ teaspoon smoked paprika

½ teaspoon freshly ground black pepper

1½ pounds white fish fillets, skin removed

2 tablespoons avocado oil or canola oil

To make the slaw

In a large glass bowl, whisk together the lime zest and juice, oil, honey, and salt. Add the cabbage and toss to coat. Cover and refrigerate.

To cook the fish

1. In a small bowl, whisk together the chili powder, cumin, salt, smoked paprika, and black pepper. Rub the spice mixture all over the fish fillets.

2. Heat the oil in a large skillet over medium-high heat. Sauté the fish fillets for 2 to 3 minutes per side, until the fish flakes easily with a fork.

To make the tacos

1. Serve the fish on corn tortillas with slaw and avocado slices.

For the tacos

12 (6-inch) corn tortillas, toasted (see Cooking Tip)

2 medium ripe avocados, pitted, peeled, and sliced

2. Store the fish in an airtight container in the refrigerator for up to 2 days. Reheat by toasting the fish under the broiler until hot. Store the slaw in a separate airtight container in the refrigerator for up to 3 days.

Variation Tip: Try salmon or chicken instead of fish. Add cilantro to the slaw for a bright flavor.

Cooking Tip: Toast the corn tortillas in a hot, dry skillet for 1 to 3 minutes per side, until slightly browned and toasted.

Nutrition Information (per serving, 2 tacos): Calories 403; Total fat 21g; Saturated fat 3g; Cholesterol 49mg; Sodium 362mg; Carbs 31g; Fiber 7g; Sugar 7g; Protein 24g

SCALLOP, BACON, AND PEA PASTA

SERVES 6 / PREP TIME: 15 TO 20 MINUTES / COOK TIME: 20 TO 25 MINUTES

This pasta is a mash-up of comfort food and ocean freshness! Bay scallops are small round scallops and are the most affordable of the scallop varieties. They are the perfect size for a pasta dish and cook up very quickly. This dish is finished with peas, Parmesan, and parsley for a light-tasting, healthy meal.

8 ounces whole-grain linguine

3 slices bacon, chopped

5 tablespoons extra-virgin olive oil, divided

1 pound bay scallops, cleaned and dried

1½ teaspoons kosher salt or sea salt, divided

½ teaspoon freshly ground black pepper, divided

6 to 7 garlic cloves, minced

4 tablespoons all-purpose flour

1½ cups unsalted seafood stock

1 cup milk

1 cup frozen spring peas

1 teaspoon dry mustard

½ teaspoon celery salt

¼ teaspoon cayenne pepper

1. Bring a large pot of water to a boil. Cook the pasta according to package directions. Reserve ¼ cup pasta water and drain the rest. Set pasta aside.

2. Heat a Dutch oven or large skillet over medium heat. Add the chopped bacon and cook for about 8 to 10 minutes, stirring frequently, until the bacon is crispy. Use a slotted spoon to transfer to a paper towel–lined plate. Discard the bacon fat.

3. Heat 3 tablespoons of olive oil in the same pot or pan over medium heat. Add the scallops, season with ½ teaspoon salt and ¼ teaspoon black pepper, and sauté for 2 to 3 minutes or until lightly browned on the outside. Remove from the pan and place on the plate with the bacon.

4. Add the remaining 2 tablespoons of olive oil and garlic to the pan and sauté for 1 to 2 minutes or until fragrant.

5. Whisk in the flour and cook for 1 to 2 minutes, until roux is lightly browned. Turn the heat to medium high and slowly whisk in the stock, bringing it to a simmer. Slowly whisk in the milk and reserved pasta liquid, then whisk constantly until thickened.

Zest and juice of ½ medium
lemon

¼ cup freshly grated
Parmesan cheese

¼ cup fresh flat-leaf Italian
parsley leaves, chopped

6. Stir in the peas, remaining 1 teaspoon salt, remaining
¼ teaspoon black pepper, dry mustard, celery salt,
cayenne pepper, lemon zest and juice, and Parmesan
cheese. Stir in the scallops, bacon, and parsley.

7. Store pasta in an airtight container in the refrigerator
for up to 2 days. Reheat by toasting under the broiler
until hot.

Variation Tip: Try a shaped pasta instead of the
linguine. Use cooked asparagus instead of peas.

Cooking Tip: Cook pasta according to package
directions to get the perfect al dente texture.

Nutrition Information (per serving): Calories 374; Total fat 16g;
Saturated fat 3g; Cholesterol 16mg; Sodium 659mg; Carbs 41g;
Fiber 5g; Sugar 6g; Protein 20g

PISTACHIO-CRUSTED SCALLOPS

SERVES 4 / PREP TIME: 10 TO 15 MINUTES / COOK TIME: 10 TO 15 MINUTES

Scallops may seem like an intimidating type of seafood to cook at home, but with a hot pan and a few other simple ingredients, it couldn't be easier to transform them into a sophisticated meal. In this recipe, the scallops are seared in hot oil and coated with a fresh-tasting mixture of pistachios, lemon zest, and salt.

½ cup shelled unsalted pistachios

Zest of 1 medium lemon

¾ teaspoon kosher salt or sea salt, divided

2 tablespoons extra-virgin olive oil

1 pound sea or diver scallops, cleaned and dried

½ teaspoon freshly ground black pepper

1. Place the pistachios in a small food processor; pulse until they resemble crumbs. Transfer the pistachio crumbs to a shallow dish and stir in the lemon zest and ¼ teaspoon of the salt. Set aside.

2. Heat the olive oil in a large skillet over medium-high heat. Season the scallops on all sides with the remaining ½ teaspoon salt and the black pepper. Add the scallops to the skillet and sauté for about 2 to 3 minutes or until browned, then flip and cook on the other side, about 1 to 2 minutes or until the scallops are slightly firm.

3. Use tongs to transfer the scallops to the dish with the pistachio crust; turn and toss the scallops until they are coated on all sides. Serve immediately.

4. Store the scallops in an airtight container in the refrigerator for up to 2 days. Reheat by toasting them under the broiler just until hot.

Variation Tip: Try almonds, walnuts, pecans, pepitas, or pine nuts instead of pistachios. Try this recipe with shrimp.

Cooking Tip: You'll know the oil is hot in the skillet when it starts to ripple.

Make It a Meal: Serve with a bowl of Tomato-Basil Bisque (page 92).

Nutrition Information (per serving): Calories 246; Total fat 18g; Saturated fat 1g; Cholesterol 36mg; Sodium 562mg; Carbs 10g; Fiber 2g; Sugar 1g; Protein 14g

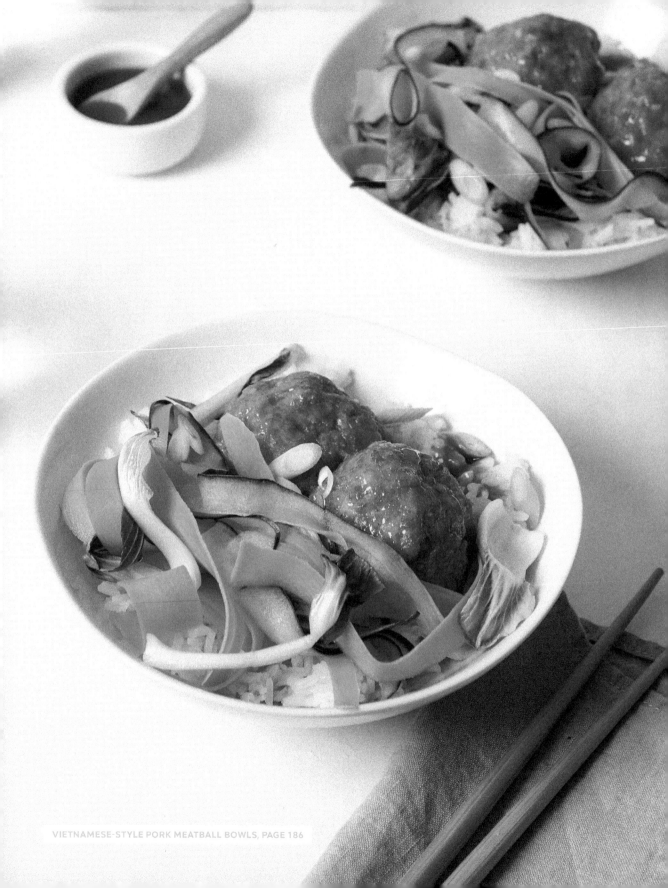

VIETNAMESE-STYLE PORK MEATBALL BOWLS, PAGE 186

CHAPTER EIGHT

Poultry and Meat Mains

GREEK-STYLE LEMON CHICKEN AND RICE SKILLET

SERVES 6 / PREP TIME: 40 TO 45 MINUTES / COOK TIME: 50 TO 60 MINUTES

This one-dish meal pairs the classic Mediterranean flavors of lemon, oregano, garlic, and olive oil with the hearty staples of chicken, spinach, and brown rice to make a complete meal. The chicken is extra delicious if marinated, but you can skip that step if you're in a bit of a hurry to get dinner on the table.

Zest and juice of 1 medium lemon

3 tablespoons extra-virgin olive oil, divided

2 tablespoons dried oregano, divided

1½ teaspoons kosher salt or sea salt, divided

½ teaspoon freshly ground black pepper, divided

2 pounds boneless, skinless chicken thighs or breasts

½ medium yellow onion, diced

3 cups baby spinach, chopped

3 to 4 garlic cloves, minced

1 cup brown rice

3 cups unsalted chicken stock

try 4 cups - rice was brittle

1. Place the lemon zest and juice, 2 tablespoons olive oil, 1 tablespoon of the oregano, ½ teaspoon of the salt, and ¼ teaspoon of the black pepper in a large sealable bag; seal and shake to mix. Add the chicken to the bag, seal, and mix to combine. Refrigerate for at least 30 minutes.

2. Heat the remaining tablespoon of the olive oil in a Dutch oven or large skillet over medium heat. Using tongs, remove the chicken from the bag and place it in the hot skillet. Set aside the marinade. Cook the chicken for 2 to 3 minutes per side or until lightly browned. Remove the chicken from the skillet and place it on a plate.

3. Add the remaining tablespoon of olive oil and the onion to the Dutch oven and sauté for 3 to 4 minutes or until the onion is soft. Stir in the spinach and garlic and cook for 2 to 3 more minutes or until the spinach is wilted.

4. Stir in the brown rice, the remaining 1 tablespoon oregano, 1 teaspoon salt, and ¼ teaspoon black pepper. Add the reserved marinade and the stock,

stir, and bring to a simmer. Cover the pan with a lid, reduce the heat to medium low, and cook for 30 to 35 minutes, stirring occasionally.

5. Add the chicken back to the pan, cover, and cook over medium heat for another 15 to 20 minutes, until the rice and chicken are cooked. Taste and adjust the seasonings, if necessary.

6. Store the chicken in an airtight container in the refrigerator for up to 4 days. Reheat it by microwaving on high for 2 to 3 minutes or until heated through.

Variation Tip: Try fresh oregano instead of dried, but use double the amount. Try farro or another ancient grain instead of brown rice.

Cooking Tip: Chicken breast can easily overcook, so check it regularly with a meat thermometer and cook it just to 165°F.

Nutrition Information (per serving): Calories 275; Total fat 12g; Saturated fat 2g; Cholesterol 73mg; Sodium 667mg; Carbs 15g; Fiber 1g; Sugar 3g; Protein 31g

MOROCCAN-STYLE CHICKEN TAGINE

SERVES 8 / PREP TIME: 45 TO 55 MINUTES / COOK TIME: 50 TO 60 MINUTES

Tagine is a North African stew or casserole that is named after the cone-shaped terra-cotta pot it is traditionally cooked in. Although this recipe isn't made that way, the spices, fresh herbs, and aromatics still provide its delicious, unique flavor. You can use garam masala or ras el hanout, both of which contain spices like coriander, cumin, cinnamon, and cardamom. This dish can be made in advance and warmed up throughout the week.

½ cup extra-virgin olive oil

Zest and juice of 2 medium lemons

1 medium yellow onion, diced

3 to 4 garlic cloves, minced

2-inch piece fresh ginger, peeled and minced

½ cup fresh cilantro leaves, chopped

½ cup fresh flat-leaf Italian parsley leaves, chopped

2 tablespoons honey

1 tablespoon garam masala or ras el hanout

2 teaspoons ground turmeric

1¾ teaspoons kosher salt or sea salt

1 teaspoon freshly ground black pepper

1. In a sealable bag, combine the olive oil, lemon zest and juice, onion, garlic, ginger, cilantro, parsley, honey, garam masala or ras el hanout, turmeric, salt, black pepper, and cayenne; seal and shake well. Add the chicken to the bag, seal, and toss to coat. Refrigerate for at least 30 minutes.

2. Preheat the oven to 400°F.

3. Transfer the chicken and marinade to a 9-by-13-inch baking dish. Add the chickpeas, spinach, green olives, and stock and toss to mix. Bake for 45 to 55 minutes or until the chicken reaches an internal temperature of 165°F. Remove the baking dish from the oven and turn the oven to broil. Stir the chicken mixture, then place it back in the oven and let it broil for 3 to 4 minutes or until browned on top.

4. Store in an airtight container in the refrigerator for up to 4 days. Reheat it by microwaving on high for 2 to 3 minutes or until heated through.

¼ teaspoon cayenne pepper

2 pounds skinless chicken pieces (bone-in or boneless)

2 (15-ounce) cans no-salt-added chickpeas, drained and rinsed

2 cups baby spinach

½ cup pitted green olives

½ cup unsalted chicken stock

Variation Tip: If you don't have garam masala or ras el hanout, use this spice combination instead: 2 teaspoons ground coriander, 1½ teaspoons ground cumin, 1½ teaspoons ground cardamom, 1 teaspoon freshly ground black pepper, ½ teaspoon ground cinnamon, and ¼ teaspoon ground cloves. Try ½ cup brown rice instead of the chickpeas. Follow the same directions, but increase the chicken broth to 1½ cups.

Cooking Tip: Adjust the cayenne pepper amount according to your spice preference. Add more if you like heat, and add less if you don't.

Nutrition Information (per serving): Calories 345; Total fat 19g; Saturated fat 3g; Cholesterol 55mg; Sodium 591mg; Carbs 18g; Fiber 6g; Sugar 6g; Protein 27g

ORANGE CHICKEN AND BROCCOLI STIR-FRY

SERVES 8 / PREP TIME: 15 TO 20 MINUTES / COOK TIME: 20 TO 25 MINUTES

Skip the takeout and opt for this healthier take on crispy orange chicken. The chicken is coated in cornstarch and pan-fried until crispy on the outside, then it's tossed with sautéed broccoli and a sauce made with fresh orange juice. Serve it with brown rice or quinoa for a flavorful and nutrition-packed dish.

For the sauce

Zest and juice of 2 medium oranges

⅓ cup honey

¼ cup low-sodium soy sauce

2 tablespoons rice wine vinegar

3 to 4 garlic cloves, minced

2-inch piece fresh ginger, peeled and minced

½ teaspoon crushed red pepper flakes

2 tablespoons cornstarch

To make the sauce

In a medium mixing bowl, whisk together the orange zest and juice, honey, soy sauce, vinegar, garlic, ginger, and red pepper flakes. Whisk in the cornstarch until it is completely dissolved. Set aside.

To make the stir-fry

1. Heat 2 tablespoons of the oil in a large skillet over medium heat. Add the broccoli and cook for 3 to 4 minutes, stirring occasionally, until slightly tender. Transfer to a plate and set aside.

2. Season the cubed chicken with the salt and black pepper. Pour the cornstarch into a large sealable plastic bag. Add the chicken, seal, and toss to coat. Heat the remaining 3 tablespoons of oil in the same large skillet over medium heat. Use tongs to transfer the coated chicken to the skillet.

3. Cook for 5 to 6 minutes, turning the cubes of chicken as they brown, until all sides are browned and the chicken is firm. Pour the orange sauce into the skillet, bring it to a simmer, and cook for 3 to 4 minutes or until the sauce is thickened. Stir in the broccoli.

For the stir-fry

5 tablespoons avocado oil or canola oil, divided

1 medium head broccoli, cut into bite-size florets

1½ pounds boneless, skinless chicken breasts, cubed

½ teaspoon kosher salt or sea salt

½ teaspoon freshly ground black pepper

¼ cup cornstarch

2 cups cooked brown rice

3 to 4 green onions, thinly sliced

4. Serve over brown rice, and garnish with green onion.

5. Store the stir-fry in an airtight container in the refrigerator for up to 4 days. Reheat it by microwaving on high for 1 to 3 minutes or until heated through.

Variation Tip: Use bottled orange juice in a pinch. Try thinly sliced flank steak instead of chicken.

Cooking Tip: Use a Microplane to grate the fresh ginger and garlic.

Nutrition Information (per serving): Calories 332; Total fat 13g; Saturated fat 1g; Cholesterol 66mg; Sodium 543mg; Carbs 33g; Fiber 3g; Sugar 14g; Protein 25g

CRISPY PARMESAN CHICKEN TENDERS

SERVES 6 / PREP TIME: 10 TO 15 MINUTES / COOK TIME: 12 TO 17 MINUTES

Chicken tenders aren't just for kids! Adults love them, too, and this version can be easily made at home in the oven with a crispy panko breading. Serve these with your favorite dipping sauce and a salad or soup to make it a complete meal.

Nonstick cooking spray

2 pounds boneless, skinless chicken breasts, cut into strips

1 teaspoon kosher salt or sea salt, divided

½ teaspoon freshly ground black pepper, divided

¾ cup all-purpose flour

4 large eggs, beaten

2 tablespoons Dijon mustard

1½ cups panko breadcrumbs

⅓ cup freshly grated Parmesan cheese

1. Preheat the oven to 400°F. Place a wire rack inside a baking sheet, and coat it with cooking spray.

2. Season the chicken breast strips with ½ teaspoon of the salt and ¼ teaspoon of the black pepper.

3. Set up 3 bowls: one with the flour, one with the beaten eggs and Dijon, and one with the panko and Parmesan. Divide the remaining ½ teaspoon salt and ¼ teaspoon black pepper among the bowls, and stir each to combine.

4. Working one at a time, dip the chicken tenders into the flour, then the egg-Dijon mixture, and then the panko-Parmesan mixture. Place the coated chicken strips on the prepared wire rack and coat them with cooking spray.

5. Bake for 12 to 17 minutes or until the chicken is firm.

6. Store the chicken tenders in an airtight container in the refrigerator for up to 4 days. Reheat by toasting them under the broiler until crispy.

Variation Tip: To make this recipe gluten free, substitute gluten-free all-purpose flour and breadcrumbs. Try turkey breast strips instead of chicken.

Cooking Tip: Use a zester to grate the Parmesan cheese.

Make It a Meal: Serve with Kale and Crispy Chickpea Caesar Salad (page 86) or Greek-Style Orzo (page 101).

Nutrition Information (per serving): Calories 295; Total fat 9g; Saturated fat 3g; Cholesterol 202mg; Sodium 661mg; Carbs 17g; Fiber 1g; Sugar 0g; Protein 37g

TURKEY-ZUCCHINI MEAT LOAF

SERVES 6 / PREP TIME: 10 TO 15 MINUTES / COOK TIME: 30 TO 40 MINUTES

Meat loaf is a family favorite, and this recipe packs in a cup of vegetables! The Parmesan cheese, Dijon mustard, Italian seasoning, garlic, and red pepper flakes provide plenty of flavor, and the homemade balsamic glaze sets it apart from other meat loaf recipes.

For the meat loaf

Nonstick cooking spray

1½ **pounds ground turkey**

1 **medium zucchini, shredded**

2 large eggs

¾ cup panko breadcrumbs

¼ cup freshly grated Parmesan cheese

3 tablespoons Dijon mustard

1 tablespoon Italian seasoning

1½ teaspoons kosher salt or sea salt

1 teaspoon garlic powder

1 teaspoon onion powder

¾ teaspoon freshly ground black pepper

½ teaspoon crushed red pepper flakes

For the glaze

½ cup balsamic vinegar

3 tablespoons dark brown sugar

To make the meat loaf

1. Preheat the oven to 375°F. Coat a 9-by-5-inch loaf pan with cooking spray.

2. In a large bowl, mix together the ground turkey, zucchini, eggs, panko breadcrumbs, Parmesan cheese, Dijon, Italian seasoning, salt, garlic powder, onion powder, black pepper, and red pepper flakes until thoroughly combined. Press the mixture evenly into the prepared bread pan. Bake for 30 to 40 minutes or until the meat loaf pulls away from the sides of the pan.

To make the glaze

1. Combine the balsamic vinegar and brown sugar in a small saucepan over medium heat. Bring the mixture to a simmer and cook for 15 to 20 minutes, stirring frequently, until thickened. Pour the mixture over the meat loaf during the last 10 minutes of cooking.

2. Remove the meat loaf from the oven and let it cool for 10 to 15 minutes, then slice and serve.

3. Store the meat loaf in an airtight container in the refrigerator for up to 4 days. Reheat it by microwaving on high for 1 to 3 minutes or until heated through.

Variation Tip: Use barbeque sauce or ketchup instead of the homemade balsamic glaze. Try this recipe with ground chicken, pork, or beef—or a mixture.

Cooking Tip: For mini versions, bake the meat loaf mixture in a muffin tin for 20 to 25 minutes.

Make It a Meal: Serve with Roasted Beet, Arugula, and Quinoa Salad (page 82) or Classic Tabbouleh (page 84).

Nutrition Information (per serving, 1 slice): Calories 240; Total fat 6g; Saturated fat 1g; Cholesterol 80mg; Sodium 536mg; Carbs 29g; Fiber 1g; Sugar 20g; Protein 24g

TURKEY SAUSAGE AND KALE BAKED ZITI

SERVES 8 / PREP TIME: 5 TO 10 MINUTES / COOK TIME: 20 TO 30 MINUTES

You can add dark leafy greens to just about any recipe, and this casserole is no exception. The kale pairs nicely with whole-grain pasta, turkey sausage, garlic, oregano, and tomato sauce, and the dish is finished off with a thin layer of gooey mozzarella cheese.

12 ounces whole-grain ziti

3 tablespoons extra-virgin olive oil

1 bunch kale, stemmed and chopped

1 pound Italian turkey sausage, casings removed

3 to 4 garlic cloves, minced

1½ tablespoons dried oregano

1 (24-ounce) jar low-sodium marinara sauce

½ teaspoon kosher salt or sea salt

½ teaspoon freshly ground black pepper

½ teaspoon crushed red pepper flakes

1 cup shredded part-skim mozzarella

1. Preheat the oven to 375°F.

2. Bring a large pot of water to a boil. Cook the pasta according to the package directions. Drain and set aside.

3. Meanwhile, heat the olive oil in a Dutch oven over medium heat. Add the kale and turkey sausage and cook, breaking up the sausage into small pieces, until the kale is wilted and the sausage is browned, about 6 to 8 minutes.

4. Stir in the garlic and oregano and sauté for 1 to 3 minutes or until the garlic is fragrant.

5. Add the marinara sauce, salt, black pepper, and red pepper flakes and bring the mixture to a simmer. Fold in the pasta and top with the mozzarella cheese. Bake uncovered for 10 to 15 minutes or until the cheese is bubbly.

6. Store the pasta in an airtight container in the refrigerator for up to 4 days. Reheat it by microwaving on high for 1 to 3 minutes or until heated through.

Variation Tip: To make it gluten-free, choose gluten-free pasta. Try any shape of whole-grain pasta.

Cooking Tip: To easily stem and chop the kale, run your hand along the stem to pull the leaves off, and then stack them in a pile, roll them up, and slice them thinly.

Make It a Meal: Serve with a green salad or a side of roasted, grilled, or steamed vegetables.

Nutrition Information (per serving): Calories 403; Total fat 18g; Saturated fat 4g; Cholesterol 61mg; Sodium 633mg; Carbs 38g; Fiber 4g; Sugar 2g; Protein 25g

TURKEY AND BLACK BEAN ENCHILADAS

SERVES 8 / PREP TIME: 15 TO 20 MINUTES / COOK TIME: 30 TO 35 MINUTES

Once you whip up a batch of the seasoning for this recipe, you can use it for any Mexican- or Southwestern-inspired cuisine. My take on enchiladas supports cognitive function because it's made with lean ground turkey, black beans, and bell peppers, all of which are loaded with vitamins and minerals.

Nonstick cooking spray

2 tablespoons avocado oil or canola oil

1 medium bell pepper, seeded and diced

½ medium yellow onion, minced

1 pound ground turkey

3 to 4 garlic cloves, minced

1½ tablespoons chili powder

2 teaspoons ground cumin

½ teaspoons kosher salt or sea salt

¾ teaspoon freshly ground black pepper

¼ teaspoon cayenne pepper

2 (15-ounce) cans no-salt-added black beans, drained and rinsed

8 (8-inch) whole-grain flour tortillas

½ cup green enchilada sauce

½ cup shredded Mexican-style cheese blend

2 medium ripe avocados, pitted, peeled, and sliced

1. Preheat the oven to 375°F. Coat a 9-by-13-inch baking dish with cooking spray.

2. Heat the oil in a large skillet over medium heat. Add the bell pepper and onion and cook for 2 to 3 minutes, until slightly soft. Add the ground turkey and sauté for 6 to 8 minutes, breaking it into small pieces with a wooden spoon. Stir in the garlic, chili powder, cumin, salt, black pepper, and cayenne. Add the black beans and ¼ cup of water and simmer for 1 to 2 minutes, until thickened.

3. Fill each tortilla with the turkey mixture. Roll up the tortillas and place them seam-side down in the baking dish. Pour the enchilada sauce over top and sprinkle with the cheese. Bake for 20 to 25 minutes or until the cheese is bubbly. Serve the enchiladas with the sliced avocado.

4. Store the enchiladas in an airtight container in the refrigerator for up to 4 days. Reheat them by microwaving on high for 1 to 3 minutes or until heated through.

Variation Tip: Make this vegetarian by swapping the meat for another can of black or pinto beans. Instead of serving this with sliced avocado, make your own guacamole with mashed avocado, chopped red onion, jalapeño, cilantro, fresh lime juice, and salt.

Make It a Meal: Serve with a green salad or a side of roasted, grilled, or steamed vegetables.

Nutrition Information (per serving, 1 enchilada): Calories 316; Total fat 16g; Saturated fat 3g; Cholesterol 15mg; Sodium 634mg; Carbs 30g; Fiber 7g; Sugar 2g; Protein 21g

SPAGHETTI SQUASH WITH TURKEY BOLOGNESE

SERVES 6 / PREP TIME: 15 TO 20 MINUTES / COOK TIME: 45 TO 60 MINUTES

Spaghetti squash is a high-fiber and gluten-free alternative to pasta. You can roast it in the oven or microwave it to create perfect spaghetti-like strands. If it gets a bit watery, use a paper towel to pat it dry. It tastes delicious with a homemade tomato sauce like this one, but if you're in a pinch, you can use a jar of low-sodium marinara or prepackaged Bolognese sauce instead of making your own.

Nonstick cooking spray

1 medium spaghetti squash, halved and seeded

3 tablespoons extra-virgin olive oil, divided

2 teaspoons kosher salt or sea salt, divided

½ medium yellow onion, peeled and diced

1½ pounds ground turkey

2 cups baby spinach or chopped kale leaves

3 to 4 garlic cloves, minced

1½ tablespoons Italian seasoning

1 (28-ounce) can no-salt-added crushed San Marzano tomatoes

¼ cup fresh basil leaves, rolled up and sliced into thin ribbons (chiffonade)

1. Preheat the oven to 375°F. Coat a 9-by-13-inch baking dish with cooking spray.

2. Place the spaghetti squash in a baking dish cut-side down, coat it with 1 tablespoon of the olive oil, and sprinkle with ½ teaspoon of the salt. Roast for 45 to 60 minutes or until fork-tender. Once the squash is cool enough to handle, use a fork to break apart the spaghetti squash flesh into strands.

3. Meanwhile, in a Dutch oven, heat the remaining 2 tablespoons of olive oil over medium heat. Add the onion and sauté for 4 to 5 minutes or until soft.

4. Add the ground turkey and spinach or kale and sauté for 6 to 8 minutes, breaking the turkey into small pieces with a wooden spoon, until the turkey is browned and the greens are wilted.

5. Stir in the garlic and Italian seasoning. Add the crushed tomatoes and basil, bring the mixture to a simmer, and cook for 20 to 25 minutes. Stir in the remaining 1½ teaspoons salt, black pepper, and sugar. Taste and adjust the seasonings, if necessary.

½ teaspoon freshly ground
black pepper

1 teaspoon sugar

¼ cup fresh flat-leaf Italian
parsley leaves, chopped

6. Serve the Bolognese sauce over the spaghetti squash, and sprinkle with the chopped parsley.

7. Store in an airtight container in the refrigerator for up to 4 days. Reheat it by microwaving on high for 1 to 3 minutes or until heated through.

Variation Tip: To make this dish vegetarian, omit the meat.

Cooking Tip: To make slicing the squash easier, cut the ends off and microwave it for 2 to 3 minutes. Let it cool, then slice it in half and scoop out the seeds.

Make It a Meal: Serve with a green salad or a side of roasted, grilled, or steamed vegetables.

Nutrition Information (per serving): Calories 262; Total fat 12g; Saturated fat 1g; Cholesterol 21mg; Sodium 486mg; Carbs 17g; Fiber 3g; Sugar 9g; Protein 32g

CRISPY PORK AND AVOCADO TACOS

SERVES 8 / PREP TIME: 5 TO 10 MINUTES / COOK TIME: 2 TO 3 HOURS

Braising means using both dry- and moist-heat cooking methods. You start by searing the pork in a bit of oil until the outside forms a crispy crust, and then you add liquid and slow cook it until it's fork-tender. This recipe has fresh orange juice, onion, garlic, and spices and makes the perfect taco filling.

3 tablespoons avocado oil or canola oil

1½ pounds pork shoulder, trimmed of fat

2 tablespoons chili powder

1 tablespoon ground cumin

1½ teaspoons kosher salt or sea salt

¾ teaspoon freshly ground black pepper

1 medium onion, thinly sliced

5 to 6 garlic cloves, sliced

Zest and juice of 2 medium oranges

16 (6-inch) corn tortillas, toasted

2 medium ripe avocados, pitted, peeled, and sliced

½ cup thinly sliced red cabbage

2 medium limes, cut into wedges

1. Heat the oil in a Dutch oven over medium-high heat. Rub the pork shoulder with chili powder, cumin, salt, and black pepper. Sear the pork shoulder for 2 to 3 minutes per side or until a thick, browned crust forms.

2. Add the onion, garlic, and orange zest and juice to the Dutch oven. Place a lid on top and reduce the heat to medium low. Simmer for 2 to 3 hours or until the pork shoulder shreds easily with a fork. If the liquid cooks off before the pork is cooked, add 1 to 2 cups of water or stock.

3. Serve the pork in toasted corn tortillas with avocado slices, cabbage, and a squeeze of lime juice.

4. Store the pork in an airtight container in the refrigerator for up to 4 days. Reheat it by microwaving on high for 1 to 3 minutes or until heated through. Assemble the tacos just before eating.

Variation Tip: Use coleslaw mix instead of sliced red cabbage. Try chicken thighs or a beef roast instead of pork.

Cooking Tip: To cook the pork in the slow cooker: Transfer the browned pork shoulder to a slow cooker. Add the onion, garlic, and orange juice and cook on high for 3 to 4 hours or on low for 6 to 8 hours.

Nutrition Information (per serving, 2 tacos): Calories 363; Total fat 18g; Saturated fat 3g; Cholesterol 56mg; Sodium 348mg; Carbs 32g; Fiber 8g; Sugar 7g; Protein 20g

VIETNAMESE-STYLE PORK MEATBALL BOWLS

SERVES 6 / PREP TIME: 15 TO 20 MINUTES / COOK TIME: 15 TO 18 MINUTES

These rice bowls feature juicy pork meatballs and a topping of quick-pickled carrots, cucumber, and bok choy. I like to batch cook the rice and meatballs on the weekend and assemble the bowls during the week for a quick meal.

For the pickled vegetables

2 medium carrots, peeled and thinly sliced

1 medium English cucumber, thinly sliced

1 small head baby bok choy, thinly sliced

2 tablespoons rice wine vinegar

¼ teaspoon kosher salt or sea salt

For the meatballs

Nonstick cooking spray

1 pound ground pork

2 large eggs

¾ cup panko breadcrumbs

3 to 4 garlic cloves, minced

1-inch piece fresh ginger, peeled and minced

2 tablespoons brown sugar

2 tablespoons soy sauce

1 teaspoon sesame oil

To make the pickled vegetables

Place the carrots, cucumber, and bok choy in a medium glass bowl; toss with the vinegar and salt. Cover and refrigerate for at least 30 minutes and up to 7 days.

To make the meatballs

1. Preheat the oven to 375°F. Place a wire rack inside a baking sheet, and coat it with cooking spray.

2. Mix the pork, eggs, panko, garlic, ginger, brown sugar, soy sauce, sesame oil, salt, and black pepper in a large mixing bowl until thoroughly combined. Form the mixture into 2-inch meatballs, and place them on the prepared wire rack. Bake for 15 to 18 minutes or until the meatballs are firm.

To assemble the bowls

1. Divide the rice among six bowls. Top with the meatballs, pickled vegetables, sriracha, and green onion. Serve immediately.

½ teaspoon kosher salt or sea salt

½ teaspoon freshly ground black pepper

For the bowls

2 cups cooked jasmine rice

1 tablespoon sriracha sauce

2 green onions, thinly sliced

2. Store the meatballs in an airtight container in the refrigerator for up to 4 days. Reheat them by microwaving on high for 1 to 3 minutes or until heated through. Store the rice, sriracha, and green onions in an airtight container in the refrigerator for up to 3 days. Store the pickled vegetables separately in an airtight container up to 7 days.

Variation Tip: Try ground turkey or chicken instead of pork. Use brown rice or quinoa instead of Jasmine rice.

Cooking Tip: Instead of baking, you can sauté the meatballs in a skillet in a bit of oil until all sides are crispy and the meatballs are firm.

Nutrition Information (per serving): Calories 328; Total fat 14g; Saturated fat 5g; Cholesterol 112mg; Sodium 595mg; Carbs 30g; Fiber 2g; Sugar 8g; Protein 19g

CUBAN-STYLE MOJO PORK TENDERLOIN

SERVES 6 / PREP TIME: 35 TO 40 MINUTES / COOK TIME: 20 TO 30 MINUTES

Generally, Cuban mojo pork is made with a shoulder or butt roast, but this is a leaner version made with pork tenderloin. It's marinated in orange and lime juices, fresh herbs, garlic, and spices, pan seared, then finished in the oven. The juices in the pan are made into a delicious sauce with just a hint of butter.

½ cup extra-virgin olive oil

Zest and juice of 2 medium oranges

Zest and juice of 6 medium limes

1 medium red bell pepper, stemmed and seeded

1 cup fresh cilantro leaves

¼ cup fresh mint leaves

2 tablespoons fresh oregano leaves

6 garlic cloves, peeled

1 tablespoon ground cumin

1½ teaspoons kosher salt or sea salt

1 teaspoon freshly ground black pepper

2 pounds pork tenderloin

1 tablespoon unsalted butter

1. In the bowl of a food processor, combine the olive oil, orange zest and juice, lime zest and juice, bell pepper, cilantro, mint, oregano, garlic, cumin, salt, and black pepper; pulse until the pepper and herbs are finely chopped, scraping the sides of the bowl as needed.

2. Pour the mixture into a gallon-sized zip-top plastic bag. Add the pork to the bag, seal, and refrigerate for at least 30 minutes or up to 24 hours.

3. Preheat the oven to 350°F.

4. Heat a large oven-safe skillet over medium high heat. Use tongs to transfer the pork to the skillet. Reserve the marinade. Sear all sides of the pork until browned and crispy.

5. Transfer the skillet to the oven, and roast the pork for 15 to 20 minutes or until the internal temperature reaches 145°F. Let the pork sit at room temperature for 5 to 10 minutes, then slice it.

6. Return the skillet to the stove over medium heat. Add the marinade and let it simmer while the pork rests, scraping up the bits on the bottom of the pan,

until it is slightly thickened. Stir in the butter until it is completely melted. Spoon the sauce over the sliced pork.

7. Store the sliced pork tenderloin in an airtight container in the refrigerator for up to 4 days. Reheat it by microwaving on high for 1 to 3 minutes or until heated through.

Cooking Tip: Because the skillet will be hot from the oven, use an oven mitt when holding the handle while making the sauce.

Variation Tip: Try this dish with beef tenderloin, or chicken or turkey breasts or thighs.

Make It a Meal: Serve with a green salad or a side of roasted, grilled, or steamed vegetables.

Nutrition Information (per serving): Calories 365; Total fat 24g; Saturated fat 5g; Cholesterol 85mg; Sodium 364mg; Carbs 8g; Fiber 2g; Sugar 2g; Protein 31g

BEEF AND SWEET POTATO SHEPHERD'S PIE

SERVES 6 / PREP TIME: 15 TO 20 MINUTES / COOK TIME: 55 TO 60 MINUTES

Shepherd's pie is traditionally made with a white potato topping, but I like to use sweet potatoes for a boost of vitamin A. The filling is made with beef, mixed vegetables, fresh thyme, and tomato paste. This dish proves that comfort food can be loaded with antioxidants!

For the sweet potato topping

3 medium sweet potatoes

¼ cup milk or plain Greek yogurt

¾ teaspoon kosher salt or sea salt

¼ teaspoon freshly ground black pepper

For the filling

2 tablespoons avocado oil or canola oil

½ medium yellow onion, diced

1 pound lean ground beef

2 cups baby spinach or chopped kale leaves

2 to 3 garlic cloves, minced

Leaves from 2 to 3 sprigs fresh thyme, chopped

1 teaspoon kosher salt or sea salt

To make the sweet potato topping

Using a fork, poke several holes in each sweet potato. Microwave the potatoes on high for 8 to 10 minutes or until fork tender. Let them cool slightly, then peel off the skins and place the flesh in a medium bowl. Add the milk or Greek yogurt, salt, and black pepper to the bowl; mash until smooth. Set aside.

To make the filling

1. Preheat the oven to 375°F.

2. Heat the oil in a Dutch oven over medium heat. Add the onion and sauté for 4 to 5 minutes, until soft.

3. Add the ground beef and spinach or kale and sauté for 6 to 8 minutes, breaking the meat into small pieces with a wooden spoon, until the beef is browned.

4. Stir in the garlic, thyme, salt, and black pepper; sauté for 1 to 3 minutes or until the garlic is fragrant.

5. Add the flour and whisk continuously until the mixture becomes bubbly. Slowly whisk in the beef stock.

6. Bring the mixture to a simmer and cook, stirring frequently, for 6 to 7 minutes.

½ teaspoon freshly ground
black pepper

3 tablespoons all-purpose
flour

2¼ cups unsalted beef stock

3 tablespoons no-salt-
added tomato paste

1 tablespoon Worcestershire
sauce

4 cups frozen mixed
vegetables

7. Reduce the heat to low and stir in the tomato paste, Worcestershire, and frozen vegetables.

To make the pie

1. Dollop the sweet potato mixture on top of the beef mixture, and spread it out in an even layer. Bake for 30 to 40 minutes or until the filling is bubbly and the potato topping is lightly browned. Remove it from the oven, let it cool slightly, and serve.

2. Store the shepherd's pie in an airtight container in the refrigerator for up to 4 days. Reheat it by microwaving on high for 2 to 3 minutes or until heated through.

Variation Tip: To make this dish dairy-free, skip the milk or Greek yogurt in the sweet potato topping. Try using ½ tablespoon of dried thyme instead of fresh. Use chopped fresh carrots and green beans instead of frozen mixed vegetables.

Nutrition Information (per serving): Calories 246; Total fat 6g; Saturated fat 1g; Cholesterol 18mg; Sodium 306mg; Carbs 32g; Fiber 5g; Sugar 9g; Protein 11g

CAULIFLOWER BEEF FRIED "RICE"

SERVES 4 / PREP TIME: 5 TO 10 MINUTES / COOK TIME: 20 TO 25 MINUTES

Cauliflower fried rice is quick, simple, and delicious. It's a complete meal with more than 6 cups of vegetables and loads of protein. Add a handful of dark leafy greens for a boost of vitamins. If you have fresh cauliflower, chop it into florets and pulse it in a food processor until it's riced. You can also typically purchase a bag of riced cauliflower in the frozen section of your grocery store, as this preparation has become quite popular recently.

For the fried "rice"

Nonstick cooking spray

4 large eggs, beaten

2 tablespoons avocado oil or canola oil

½ medium yellow onion, diced

1 pound lean ground beef

2 to 3 garlic cloves, minced

2-inch piece fresh ginger, peeled and minced

4 cups riced cauliflower

2 cups frozen peas and carrots

To make the fried "rice"

1. Heat a large nonstick skillet over medium heat. Coat the skillet with cooking spray, then add the beaten eggs. Use a flat spatula to scramble the eggs just until they're cooked through, and transfer them to a plate.

2. Heat the oil in the same skillet over medium heat. Add the onion and sauté for 4 to 5 minutes or until soft. Add the ground beef and sauté for 6 to 8 minutes, breaking it into small pieces with a wooden spoon, until the meat is browned. Add the garlic and ginger and sauté for 1 to 3 minutes or until fragrant. Stir in the riced cauliflower and peas and carrots; sauté for 4 to 5 minutes or until the vegetables are soft.

To make the sauce

1. In a small bowl, whisk together the soy sauce, lime zest and juice, honey, sesame oil, and sriracha. Stir the sauce into the riced cauliflower and bring the mixture

For the sauce

2 tablespoons low-sodium
  soy sauce

Zest and juice of
  ½ medium lime

1 tablespoon honey

2 teaspoons sesame oil

2 teaspoons sriracha sauce

2 green onions, thinly sliced

to a simmer. Cook until the sauce thickens, then fold in the scrambled eggs. Serve in bowls, topped with sliced green onion.

2. Store in an airtight container in the refrigerator for up to 4 days. Reheat it by microwaving on high for 1 to 2 minutes or until heated through.

Variation Tip: Use cooked brown rice instead of riced cauliflower. Swap out the beef for ground pork, chicken, or turkey.

Nutrition Information (per serving): Calories 313; Total fat 16g; Saturated fat 4g; Cholesterol 211mg; Sodium 564mg; Carbs 23g; Fiber 5g; Sugar 8g; Protein 17g

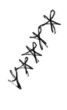

BEEF AND RICE FAJITA CASSEROLE

SERVES 6 / PREP TIME: 15 TO 20 MINUTES / COOK TIME: 30 TO 40 MINUTES

To have this casserole ready in no time, you can batch cook the rice on the weekend and add it with the rest of the ingredients just before baking. The onions, peppers, and beef could also be prepped in advance.

Nonstick cooking spray

2 tablespoons avocado oil or canola oil

1 medium red onion, diced

1 medium red bell pepper, seeded and diced

1 medium green bell pepper, seeded and diced

1½ pounds lean ground beef

3 to 4 garlic cloves, minced

2 tablespoons chili powder

2 teaspoons ground cumin

1 teaspoon smoked paprika

1 teaspoon kosher salt or sea salt

½ teaspoon freshly ground black pepper

3 cups cooked brown rice

½ cup green enchilada sauce

1 cup shredded Mexican-style cheese blend

½ cup plain Greek yogurt

½ cup fresh cilantro leaves, chopped

1. Preheat the oven to 375°F. Coat a 9-by-13-inch baking dish with cooking spray. Set it aside.

2. Heat the oil in a large skillet over medium heat. Add the onion and bell peppers, and sauté for 4 to 5 minutes or until soft. Add the ground beef and sauté for 6 to 8 minutes, breaking it into small pieces with a wooden spoon, until the beef is browned. Add the garlic and sauté for 1 to 3 minutes, until fragrant. Stir in the chili powder, cumin, smoked paprika, salt, and black pepper. Add the rice and enchilada sauce; stir until well combined.

3. Transfer the mixture to the prepared baking dish, and top with the shredded cheese. Bake for 25 to 30 minutes or until the cheese is bubbly and browned. Remove the casserole from the oven; serve hot with Greek yogurt and cilantro.

4. Store the casserole in an airtight container in the refrigerator for up to 4 days. Reheat it by microwaving on high for 1 to 2 minutes or until heated through.

Variation Tip: Use 3 tablespoons of low-sodium taco seasoning instead of the chili powder, cumin, smoked paprika, salt, and black pepper. Swap out the ground beef for thinly sliced beef flank steak.

Cooking Tip: You can use plain Greek yogurt in place of sour cream in most recipes.

Nutrition Information (per serving): Calories 264; Total fat 9g; Saturated fat 2g; Cholesterol 26mg; Sodium 401mg; Carbs 32g; Fiber 5g; Sugar 5g; Protein 11g

GREEK-STYLE LAMB GYROS

SERVES 6 / PREP TIME: 15 TO 20 MINUTES / COOK TIME: 20 TO 30 MINUTES

Traditional gyro meat is cooked on a rotisserie, and because most of us don't have that equipment at home, this version calls for ground lamb combined with mouthwatering spices. It cooks up in minutes and is served on fluffy pita bread with crisp cucumber slices, Greek yogurt, and feta cheese.

2 tablespoons avocado oil or canola oil

½ medium yellow onion, diced

1 pound ground lamb

3 to 4 garlic cloves, minced

½ tablespoon ground coriander

½ tablespoon ground cumin

2 teaspoons dried oregano

1 teaspoon kosher salt or sea salt

½ teaspoon freshly ground black pepper

¼ teaspoon ground cinnamon

¼ teaspoon cayenne pepper (optional)

6 whole-grain pitas

½ medium English cucumber, thinly sliced

½ cup plain Greek yogurt

¼ cup crumbled feta cheese (optional)

1. Heat the oil in a skillet over medium heat. Add the onion and sauté for 4 to 5 minutes or until soft. Add the ground lamb and sauté for 6 to 8 minutes, breaking it into small pieces with a wooden spoon, until the lamb is browned. Add the garlic and sauté for 1 to 2 minutes or until fragrant. Stir in the coriander, cumin, oregano, salt, black pepper, cinnamon, cayenne (if using), and ¼ cup of water. Bring the mixture to a simmer and cook just until it thickens, 3 to 5 minutes.

2. Spoon the meat mixture into the pitas, and layer with cucumber, yogurt, and feta cheese, if using.

3. Store the meat mixture in an airtight container in the refrigerator for up to 4 days. Reheat it by microwaving on high for 1 to 2 minutes or until heated through.

Variation Tip: Swap out the lamb for ground beef, chicken, or turkey.

Cooking Tip: If there is excess fat in the pan after cooking the lamb, drain it out before you add the garlic.

Make It a Meal: Serve with a green salad or a side of roasted, grilled, or steamed vegetables.

Nutrition Information (per serving): Calories 375; Total fat 18g; Saturated fat 5g; Cholesterol 61mg; Sodium 482mg; Carbs 35g; Fiber 4g; Sugar 2g; Protein 21g

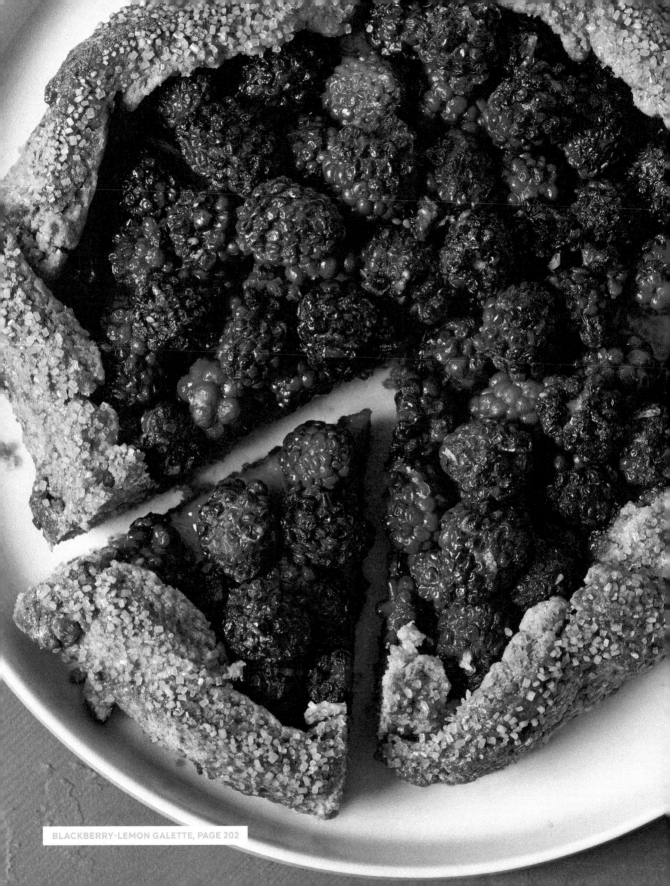

BLACKBERRY-LEMON GALETTE, PAGE 202

CHAPTER NINE

Sweet Treats

SNICKERDOODLE WHITE BEAN BLONDIES

SERVES 8 / PREP TIME: 10 TO 15 MINUTES / COOK TIME: 30 TO 35 MINUTES

These blondies are made with classic snickerdoodle flavors—vanilla, cinnamon and sugar—but they're made healthier with a base of puréed chickpeas and whole wheat flour. I promise you won't even realize there are beans in this recipe!

1 (15-ounce) can no-salt-added chickpeas, drained and rinsed

2 large eggs

¾ cup packed dark brown sugar

3 tablespoons avocado oil or canola oil

1½ tablespoons pure vanilla extract

½ teaspoon kosher salt or sea salt

½ cup whole wheat flour or whole wheat pastry flour

2 tablespoons granulated sugar

1 tablespoon ground cinnamon

1. Preheat the oven to 350°F. Line an 8-inch square baking dish with a long piece of parchment paper. The paper should hang over the edges of the dish, leaving "handles" on either side to help you lift out the blondies after baking.

2. In the bowl of a food processor, combine the chickpeas, eggs, brown sugar, oil, vanilla extract, and salt. Process until smooth, scraping down the sides of the bowl with a spatula as needed. Add the flour and pulse until just combined.

3. Transfer the mixture to the prepared baking dish, and spread it out evenly.

4. In a small bowl, whisk together the granulated sugar and cinnamon. Sprinkle the mixture evenly over the batter. Bake for 30 to 35 minutes or until a toothpick inserted into the center comes out clean. Remove the baking dish from the oven, let the blondies cool, and then use the parchment to lift the blondies out of the dish. Cut into eight squares and serve.

5. Store the blondies in an airtight bag or container at room temperature for up to 7 days.

Variation Tip: Use any cooked white beans. Fold dark chocolate chips or raisins into the batter before baking.

Cooking Tip: Be sure to purée the chickpeas until they are very smooth, to avoid clumps of beans in the final product.

Nutrition Information (per serving, 1 blondie): Calories 203; Total fat 7g; Saturated fat 1g; Cholesterol 47mg; Sodium 106mg; Carbs 30g; Fiber 4g; Sugar 22g; Protein 5g

BLACKBERRY-LEMON GALETTE

SERVES 8 / PREP TIME: 20 TO 25 MINUTES / COOK TIME: 40 TO 45 MINUTES

A galette is like an open-faced pie. The crust is crispy, the berry filling is both sweet and tart, and when served with a scoop of vanilla ice cream, it's heaven. It is easier to make than pie, and the charm of it is that it's rustic, so you don't have to stress about making it look perfect. It's just scrumptious!

For the crust

Nonstick cooking spray

⅔ **cup avocado oil or canola oil**

1 large egg

3 tablespoons granulated sugar

2¼ **cups whole wheat flour or whole wheat pastry flour**

½ teaspoon kosher salt or sea salt

2 tablespoons milk

For the filling

2½ **cups frozen or fresh blackberries**

⅓ cup granulated sugar

Zest and juice of ½ medium lemon

1½ tablespoons cornstarch

For the gallette

1 large egg, beaten

½ tablespoon turbinado sugar

2 cups vanilla frozen yogurt or ice cream (optional)

To make the crust

1. Preheat the oven to 400°F. Coat a rimmed baking sheet with cooking spray or line with parchment paper.

2. In a medium bowl, whisk together the oil, egg, and sugar until fluffy. Stir in the flour and salt. Add the milk and stir until the dough comes together into pea-size pieces.

3. Transfer the mixture to a lightly floured cutting board and sprinkle with additional flour. Roll out the dough to a ½-inch circle, then transfer it to the prepared baking sheet.

To make the filling

In another medium mixing bowl, stir together the berries, sugar, lemon zest and juice, and cornstarch until combined.

To make the galette

1. Spoon the berry mixture onto the dough circle, leaving a 2-inch border around the edge. Fold the dough edges up and over the edges of the filling. Brush the beaten egg over the dough edges and sprinkle with the turbinado sugar.

2. Bake for 40 to 45 minutes, or until the crust is browned and crisp and the filling is bubbly. Remove the galette from the oven, let it cool, and then slice it into eight wedges. Serve with vanilla frozen yogurt or ice cream, if desired.

3. Store the galette in an airtight container in the refrigerator for up to 3 days.

Variation Tip: Whole wheat all-purpose flour can be used instead of whole wheat pastry flour. Try mixed berries instead of blackberries.

Cooking Tip: If the dough feels a bit wet, add a little extra flour until it has the texture of pie dough.

Nutrition Information (per serving, 1 slice): Calories 358; Total fat 20g; Saturated fat 3g; Cholesterol 47mg; Sodium 90mg; Carbs 40g; Fiber 7g; Sugar 12g; Protein 6g

PUMPKIN OATMEAL RAISIN COOKIES

MAKES 20 COOKIES / PREP TIME: 10 TO 15 MINUTES / COOK TIME: 8 TO 11 MINUTES

These fluffy cookies are so tasty that you'll want to enjoy them year-round—not just in the fall. Pumpkin purée is a great source of beta carotene, and the oats have lots of soluble fiber, which is great for heart health. I like to use dark brown sugar because it has a rich, concentrated molasses flavor, so I don't have to use as much of it as I would granulated sugar.

2 cups whole wheat flour or whole wheat pastry flour

1 cup old-fashioned rolled oats

1 teaspoon baking powder

1 teaspoon baking soda

2 teaspoons ground cinnamon

1 teaspoon pumpkin pie spice

½ teaspoon kosher salt or sea salt

¾ cup packed dark brown sugar

¼ cup unsalted butter, softened

2 large eggs

1½ cups pumpkin purée

2 teaspoons pure vanilla extract

¾ cup raisins

1. Preheat the oven to 350°F. Line a baking sheet with parchment paper.

2. In a medium bowl, whisk together the flour, oats, baking powder, baking soda, cinnamon, pumpkin pie spice, and salt.

3. In another medium bowl, use a hand mixer to beat together the brown sugar and butter until fluffy. Beat in the eggs, then the pumpkin purée, and then the vanilla extract until combined. Slowly beat in the dry ingredients until just combined. Fold in the raisins with a wooden spoon or rubber spatula.

4. Use a medium cookie scoop to scoop balls of the dough into 2-inch balls, and line them up on the prepared baking sheet, 1 to 2 inches apart. Bake for 8 to 11 minutes or until the cookies are just starting to brown on the edges. Remove the cookies from the oven; let them cool slightly before serving.

5. Store the cookies in an airtight plastic bag or container at room temperature for up to 7 days.

Variation Tip: Use gluten-free all-purpose flour for gluten-free cookies. Try puréed sweet potato instead of pumpkin.

Cooking Tip: For fluffier cookies, refrigerate the cookie dough for 30 minutes before scooping and baking. If you don't have a cookie scoop, use a small ice cream scoop or a regular spoon.

Nutrition Information (per serving, 1 cookie): Calories 154; Total fat 4g; Saturated fat 2g; Cholesterol 25mg; Sodium 123mg; Carbs 30g; Fiber 2g; Sugar 17g; Protein 3g

CHOCOLATE AVOCADO MOUSSE

SERVES 8 / PREP TIME: 10 TO 15 MINUTES / CHILLING TIME: 30 MINUTES OR MORE

Avocado adds a creamy richness to this mousse, and it provides monounsaturated fats that are good for your heart. Dark chocolate also has antioxidants—and the darker, the better. Serve this mousse with brain-healthy berries and sprigs of mint for a luxurious, fancy-looking dessert.

½ cup dark chocolate chips

½ cup milk

2 medium ripe avocados, pitted and peeled

½ cup pure maple syrup, honey, or granulated sugar

1 teaspoon pure vanilla extract

¼ teaspoon kosher salt or sea salt

1 cup fresh berries

8 small sprigs fresh mint (optional)

1. Place the chocolate chips in a glass bowl and microwave in 30-second increments, stirring in between, until melted.

2. Transfer the melted chocolate to a blender and add the milk; avocado; maple syrup; honey, or sugar; vanilla extract; and salt. Purée until very smooth, scraping down the sides of the pitcher as needed. Transfer the mixture to a bowl; cover and refrigerate for at least 30 minutes.

3. Serve the chilled mousse with fresh berries and mint sprigs, if desired.

4. Store the mousse in an airtight container in the refrigerator for up to 3 days.

Variation Tip: Use cow's, almond, soy, or coconut milk. Try chocolate milk instead of regular milk for a bolder chocolate flavor.

Cooking Tip: Be sure the avocados are ripe. They should feel soft, and the stem ends should fall off easily when plucked.

Nutrition Information (per serving): Calories 203; Total fat 10g; Saturated fat 4g; Cholesterol 3mg; Sodium 56mg; Carbs 29g; Fiber 4g; Sugar 21g; Protein 1g

MINI STRAWBERRY CHEESECAKE PARFAITS

SERVES 8 / PREP TIME: 10 TO 15 MINUTES

Not only are berries great for brain health, they're also sweet, juicy, and the stars of this deliciously creamy cheesecake parfait. The crust is made of graham crackers, crushed almonds, and just enough butter to give it that classic flavor.

6 graham cracker sheets

¼ **cup sliced unsalted almonds**

2 tablespoons melted unsalted butter

8 ounces low-fat cream cheese, softened

½ cup vanilla Greek yogurt

¼ cup sugar

2 teaspoons pure vanilla extract

1½ **cups strawberries, hulled and sliced**

1. Place the graham crackers, almonds, and butter in a small food processor; pulse until the mixture is coarsely ground. Divide half of the mixture among eight mini dessert glasses. Set the remaining crust mixture aside.

2. Place the cream cheese in a medium bowl, and use a hand mixer to beat it until it is very smooth. Add the yogurt, sugar, and vanilla extract and beat until fluffy. Divide the mixture among the dessert glasses, on top of the crust. Sprinkle the remaining crust on top of the cheesecake mixture. Top each glass with sliced strawberries and serve.

3. Store the cheesecakes in an airtight container in the refrigerator for up to 2 days.

Variation Tip: Use coconut oil instead of butter. Use mascarpone instead of cream cheese.

Cooking Tip: If you don't have a food processor, place the graham crackers in a zip-top plastic bag and crush them with a rolling pin.

Nutrition Information (per serving, 1 parfait): Calories 169; Total fat 10g; Saturated fat 5g; Cholesterol 24mg; Sodium 141mg; Carbs 16g; Fiber 1g; Sugar 11g; Protein 5g

CINNAMON-PEAR SNACK CAKE

SERVES 8 / PREP TIME: 10 TO 15 MINUTES / COOK TIME: 45 TO 55 MINUTES

I'm not sure there's a specific definition for a snack cake, but in my book, it's a cake that's packed with nutritious ingredients like oats, fruit, and spices. This version features pears and cinnamon, and the walnuts add a nutty flavor, crunch, and a dose of omega-3s. It becomes breakfast when it's drizzled with a little maple syrup.

1 cup whole wheat flour or whole wheat pastry flour

1 cup old-fashioned rolled oats

2 teaspoons baking powder

1 teaspoon ground cinnamon

½ teaspoon kosher salt or sea salt

½ teaspoon ground ginger

1 cup unsweetened applesauce

¼ cup avocado oil or canola oil

¾ cup packed dark brown sugar

1 large egg

2 teaspoons pure vanilla extract

1 medium Bartlett pear, halved, cored, and diced (skin on)

½ cup chopped unsalted walnuts or pecans, divided

1. Preheat the oven to 350°F. Line a 9-inch square baking dish with a long piece of parchment paper, and let the paper hang over the edges.

2. In a medium bowl, whisk together the flour, oats, baking powder, cinnamon, salt, and ginger.

3. In another medium bowl, use a hand mixer to beat together the applesauce, oil, and brown sugar until fluffy. Add the egg and vanilla extract and beat until well combined. Slowly beat in the dry ingredients until just combined. Fold in the diced pears and half of the walnuts.

4. Transfer the batter to the prepared baking dish, and spread it out evenly. Sprinkle the remaining walnuts on top, and gently press them into the batter. Bake for 35 to 45 minutes or until a toothpick inserted into

the center comes out clean. Remove the cake from the oven, let it cool, and then use the parchment paper "handles" to lift it out of the baking dish. Cut the cake into eight squares and serve.

5. Store the snack cake in sealed plastic bag or container at room temperature for up to 7 days.

Variation Tip: Try ground oats or oat flour instead of whole wheat flour. Try apples instead of pears—or both!

Cooking Tip: Take care not to overmix the batter. Once the ingredients are mixed, it's ready to go in the oven. Overmixing can make for a dry, dense cake.

Nutrition Information (per serving, 1 square): Calories 208; Total fat 11g; Saturated fat 1g; Cholesterol 16mg; Sodium 134mg; Carbs 28g; Fiber 4g; Sugar 15g; Protein 3g

CARROT CAKE-WALNUT MUFFINS

MAKES 12 MUFFINS / PREP TIME: 10 TO 15 MINUTES / COOK TIME: 20 TO 25 MINUTES

Carrot cake is a guaranteed crowd favorite. I've captured the classic carrot cake flavors in these nutrient-dense muffins, which are packed with carrots, crushed pineapple, walnuts, and coconut. They can be prepped ahead of time, frozen, and thawed out as needed. That's if you don't scarf them down straight out of the oven!

1 cup whole wheat flour or whole wheat pastry flour

1 cup old-fashioned rolled oats

1 teaspoon baking powder

1 teaspoon ground cinnamon

½ teaspoon kosher salt or sea salt

½ cup packed dark brown sugar

⅓ **cup avocado oil or canola oil**

1 large egg

½ cup milk

1 teaspoon pure vanilla extract

¼ cup crushed pineapple, drained

2 medium carrots, grated (1 cup)

½ **cup chopped unsalted walnuts, divided**

¼ cup unsweetened coconut flakes, divided

1. Preheat the oven to 350°F. Line a 12-cup muffin tin with muffin liners.

2. In a medium bowl, whisk together the flour, oats, baking powder, cinnamon, and salt.

3. In a separate medium bowl, use a hand mixer to beat together the brown sugar and oil until fluffy. Beat in the egg, then the milk, and then the vanilla extract until combined. Slowly beat in the dry ingredients until just incorporated.

4. Using a wooden spoon or rubber spatula, fold in the crushed pineapple, grated carrots, ¼ cup of the chopped walnuts, and 2 tablespoons of the shredded coconut.

5. Scoop the batter into the muffin wells, filling each well almost to the top. Top each with some of the remaining chopped walnuts and coconut, gently pressing them into the batter.

6. Bake for 18 to 22 minutes or until a toothpick inserted into the center of a muffin comes out clean. Remove the muffins from the oven and let them cool.

7. Store the muffins in an airtight plastic bag or container at room temperature for up to 5 days.

Variation Tip: Leave out the coconut, if you're not a fan. Fold ½ cup raisins into the batter, along with the pineapple and carrots.

Cooking Tip: The quickest way to grate carrots is in a food processor fitted with a shredding attachment.

Nutrition Information (per serving, 1 muffin): Calories 190; Total fat 11g; Saturated fat 2g; Cholesterol 16mg; Sodium 104mg; Carbs 21g; Fiber 2g; Sugar 10g; Protein 3g

CRUSTLESS APPLE PIES

SERVES 8 / PREP TIME: 15 TO 20 MINUTES / COOK TIME: 30 TO 35 MINUTES

Or should they be called individual apple crisps? No matter what you call them, you'll love them! In this recipe, baked apple halves are stuffed with a cinnamon-maple oat crumble that's warm, cozy, and delicious. Serve them as is or à la mode for the perfect dessert.

4 medium Granny Smith, Honeycrisp, or Braeburn apples, halved lengthwise (skin-on)

4 tablespoons melted unsalted butter, divided

4 tablespoons pure maple syrup, divided

1 cup old-fashioned rolled oats

½ cup chopped unsalted walnuts or pecans

1 teaspoon ground cinnamon

2 cups vanilla frozen yogurt or ice cream (optional)

1. Preheat the oven to 375°F.

2. Trim small slices off the skin sides of the apple halves (so they lay flat in the baking dish, flesh-side up). Use a melon baller to scoop out the apple cores. Place the apple halves in a baking dish, flesh-sides up. Brush them with 1 tablespoon of the melted butter. Bake for 20 to 25 minutes or until the apples are starting to soften.

3. Meanwhile, in a medium bowl, stir together the remaining 3 tablespoons of melted butter, 2 tablespoons of the maple syrup, and the oats, nuts, and cinnamon until combined. Spoon the mixture into the wells of the apples, return them to the oven, and bake for an additional 10 minutes, until the oats are toasted and the apples are fork tender.

4. Drizzle the apples with the remaining 2 tablespoons of maple syrup, and serve with vanilla frozen yogurt or ice cream, if desired.

5. Store the baked apples in an airtight container in the refrigerator for up to 3 days. Reheat them by microwaving on high for 1 to 3 minutes until heated through.

Variation Tip: Use oil instead of butter. In the summertime, use peaches instead of apples.

Cooking Tip: For optimal texture and fiber, leave the skin on the apples when making desserts.

Nutrition Information (per serving, 1 baked apple half): Calories 189; Total fat 10g; Saturated fat 4g; Cholesterol 15mg; Sodium 2mg; Carbs 26g; Fiber 4g; Sugar 15g; Protein 2g

Lifestyle Tracker

Use this chart to help you keep up with all aspects of the MIND diet, from what you eat to the intellectually stimulating activities you take part in on a daily and weekly basis. You can photocopy the blank meal plan or download it from CallistoMediaBooks.com/MINDDiet.

Sample MIND Diet Lifestyle Tracker

	Food	Exercise	Sleep	Stress Reduction	Intellectual Pursuits
MON	Ate ½ cup cooked spinach, ½ cup cooked root vegetables, ½ cup cooked quinoa, 1 oz. almonds, 4 oz. salmon.	Walked 30 minutes.	Moved my electronics out of the bedroom and got 8 hours of sleep.		Listened to an audio-book while I walked.
TUES	Ate 1 cup spring mix, ½ cup cooked root vegetables, 1 oz. walnuts, ½ cup beans.	Took a 30-minute yoga class.	Slept 7–8 hours.	Talked to my daughter on the phone.	
WED	Ate ½ cup cooked spinach, ½ cup cooked asparagus, 2 corn tortillas, 1 oz. almonds, ½ cup beans.	Walked 30 minutes, did 30 minutes of strength training.	Slept 7–8 hours.		Played guitar with friends.
THURS	Ate ½ cup cooked Swiss chard, ½ cup cooked asparagus, 1 oz. walnuts.	Took a 30-minute dance class.	Slept 7–8 hours.	Took a bath.	
FRI	Ate ½ cup cooked spinach, 1 cup raw baby carrots, 1 oz. almonds, 4 oz. turkey.		Slept 7–8 hours.	Went for a walk in the park.	Read a book.
SAT	Ate ½ cup cooked kale, 1 cup cooked zucchini, 4 oz. turkey, ½ cup beans.	Went on a 30-minute bike ride.	Slept 7–8 hours.		Did a cross-word puzzle.
SUN	Ate ½ cup cooked Swiss chard, ½ cup cooked cauliflower, 1 whole grain baguette.	Played with my grandkids in the park.	Slept 7–8 hours.		Went to dinner with my family.

MIND Diet Lifestyle Tracker

	Food	Exercise	Sleep	Stress Reduction	Intellectual Pursuits
MON					
TUES					
WED					
THURS					
FRI					
SAT					
SUN					

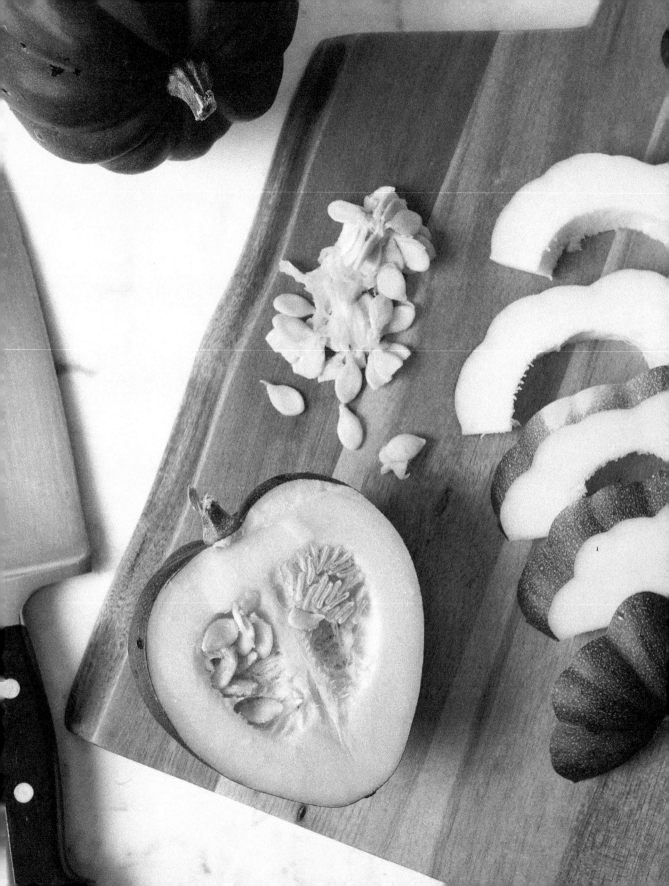

Measurement Conversions

Volume Equivalents (Liquid)

US Standard	US Standard (ounces)	Metric (approximate)
2 tablespoons	1 fl. oz.	30 mL
¼ cup	2 fl. oz.	60 mL
½ cup	4 fl. oz.	120 mL
1 cup	8 fl. oz.	240 mL
1½ cups	12 fl. oz.	355 mL
2 cups or 1 pint	16 fl. oz.	475 mL
4 cups or 1 quart	32 fl. oz.	1 L
1 gallon	128 fl. oz.	4 L

Oven Temperatures

Fahrenheit	Celsius (approximate)
250°F	120°C
300°F	150°C
325°F	165°C
350°F	180°C
375°F	190°C
400°F	200°C
425°F	220°C
450°F	230°C

Volume Equivalents (Dry)

US Standard	Metric (approximate)
⅛ teaspoon	0.5 mL
¼ teaspoon	1 mL
½ teaspoon	2 mL
¾ teaspoon	4 mL
1 teaspoon	5 mL
1 tablespoon	15 mL
¼ cup	59 mL
⅓ cup	79 mL
½ cup	118 mL
⅔ cup	156 mL
¾ cup	177 mL
1 cup	235 mL
2 cups or 1 pint	475 mL
3 cups	700 mL
4 cups or 1 quart	1 L

Weight Equivalents

US Standard	Metric (approximate)
½ ounce	15 g
1 ounce	30 g
2 ounces	60 g
4 ounces	115 g
8 ounces	225 g
12 ounces	340 g
16 ounces or 1 pound	455 g

References

Ahlskog, Eric, Yonas Geda, Neill Graff-Radford, and Ronald Petersen. "Physical Exercise as a Preventive or Disease-Modifying Treatment of Dementia and Brain Aging." *Mayo Clinic Proceedings*. 2011 Sep; 86(9): 876-884.

Alzheimer's Association. "Why Get Checked?" Accessed November 24, 2018. https://www.alz.org /alzheimers-dementia/diagnosis/why-get-checked.

Appel, L.J., et al. "A Clinical Trial of the Effects of Dietary Patterns on Blood Pressure." *New England Journal of Medicine*. 1997 Apr; 336(16): 1117-24.

Bennett, David, Julie Schneider, Aron Buchman, Lisa Barnes, Patricia Boyle, and Robert Wilson. "Overview and Findings from the Rush Memory and Aging Project." *Current Alzheimer's Research*. 2012 Jul 1; 9(6): 646–663.

Boyle, P.A., A.S. Buchman, R.S. Wilson, L. Yu, J.A. Schneider, and D.A. Bennett. "Effect of Purpose In Life on the Relation Between Alzheimer Disease Pathologic Changes on Cognitive Function in Advanced Age." *Archives in General Psychiatry*. 2012 May; 69(5): 499-505.

Brown, Benjamin. "Reversal of Alzheimer's Disease and Optimization of Brain Health with Orthomolecular Medicine." *Journal of Orthomolecular Medicine*. 2017 Oct; 32(5).

Cahill, L.E., S.E. Chiuve, Q. Sun, W.C. Willett, F.B. Hu, and E.B. Rimm. "Fried-Food Consumption and Risk of Type 2 Diabetes and Coronary Artery Disease: A Prospective Study in 2 Cohorts of US Women and Men." *American Journal of Clinical Nutrition*. 2014 Aug; 100(2): 667-75.

Cassidy, Aedin, Kenneth Mukamal, Lydia Liu, Mary Franz, Heather Eliassen, and Eric Rimm. "High Anthocyanin Intake Associated with a Reduced Risk of Myocardial Infarction in Young and Middle-Aged Women." *Circulation*. 2013 Jan; 127(2): 188-196.

Cedars-Sinai. "Subjective Cognitive Impairment (SCI)." Accessed December 3, 2018. https://www .cedars-sinai.edu/Patients/Health-Conditions/Subjective-Cognitive-Impairment-SCI.aspx.

Colcombe, S.J., et al. "Aerobic Exercise Training Increases Brain Volume in Aging Humans." *The Journals of Gerontology*. 2006 Nov; 61(11): 1166-70.

Devore, E.E., J.H. Kang, M.M. Breteler, and F. Grodstein. "Dietary Intakes of Berries and Flavonoids in Relation to Cognitive Decline." *Annals of Neurology*. 2012 Jul; 72(1): 135-43.

Estruch, R., et al. "Primary Prevention of Cardiovascular Disease with a Mediterranean Diet." *New England Journal of Medicine*. 2014 Feb; 370(9): 886.

Feart, C., et al. "Plasma Carotenoids are Inversely Associated with Dementia Risk in an Elderly French Cohort." *The Journals of Gerontology*. 2016 May; 71(5): 683-8.

Forbes, Scott, Jayna Holroyd-Leduc, Marc Poulin, and David Hogan. "Effect of Nutrients, Dietary Supplements and Vitamins on Cognition: A Systematic Review and Meta-Analysis of Randomized Controlled Trials." *Canadian Geriatrics Journal*. 2015 Dec; 18(4): 231-245.

Fratiglioni, Laura, Stephanie Paillard-Borg, and Bengt Winblad. "An Active and Socially Integrated Lifestyle in Late Life Might Protect Against Dementia." *The Lancet Neurology*. 2004 Jun; 3(6): 343-353.

Garcia, Angeles and Katherine Zanibbi. "Homocysteine and Cognitive Function in Elderly People." *Canadian Medical Association Journal*. 2004 Oct; (8)171.

Goldstein, I.B., G. Bartzokis, D. Guthrie, and D. Shapiro. "Ambulatory Blood Pressure and Brain Atrophy in the Healthy Elderly." *Neurology*. 2002 Sep; 59(5): 713-9.

Gomez-Pinilla. "Brain Foods: The Effects of Nutrients on Brain Function." *Nature Reviews Neurology*. 2008 Jul; 9(7): 568–578.

Grodstein, F., J.H. Kang, R.J. Glynn, N.R. Cook, and J.M. Gaziano. "A Randomized Trial of Beta Carotene Supplementation and Cognitive Function in Med: The Physician's Health Study II." *Archives of Internal Medicine*. 2007 Nov; 167(20): 2184-90.

Hardman, Roy, Greg Kennedy, Helen Macpherson, Scholey Pipingas, and Andrew Pipingas. "Adherence to a Mediterranean-Style Diet and Effects on Cognition in Adults: A Qualitative Evaluation And Systematic Review Of Longitudinal And Prospective Trials." *Frontiers in Nutrition*. 2016 July; 3: 22.

Harvard T.H. Chan School of Public Health. "Three of the B Vitamins: Folate, Vitamin B6, and Vitamin B12." Accessed November 22, 2018. https://www.hsph.harvard.edu/nutritionsource /what-should-you-eat/vitamins/vitamin-b.

James, B.D., R.S. Wilson, L.L. Barnes, and D.A. Bennett. "Late-Life Social Activity and Cognitive Decline in Old Age." *Journal of International Neuropsychological Society*. 2011 Nov; 17(6): 998-1005.

Ju, Yo-El, Brendan Lucey, and David Holtzman. "Sleep and Alzheimer Disease Pathology—a Bidirectional Relationship." *Nature Reviews Neurology*. 2014; 10: 115-119.

Kang, Jae, Alberto Ascherio, and Francine Grodstein. "Fruit and Vegetable Consumption and Cognitive Decline in Aging Women." *Annals of Neurology*. 2005 Apr; 57(5).

Katz, Mindy, et al. "Influence on Perceived Stress on Incident Amnestic Mild Cognitive Impairment: Results From the Einstein Aging Study." *Alzheimer's Disease & Associated Disorders*. 2017 Apr-Jun; 30(2): 93-98.

Kruman, Inna, et al. "Folic Acid Deficiency and Homocysteine Impair DNA Repair in Hippocampal Neurons and Sensitize Them to Amyloid Toxicity in Experimental Models of Alzheimer's Disease." *Journal of Neuroscience*. 2002 Mar; 22(5): 1752-1762.

La Fata, Giorgio, Peter Weber, and M. Hasan Mohajeri. "Effects of Vitamin E on Cognitive Performance During Ageing and in Alzheimer's Disease." *Nutrients*. 2014 Dec; 6(12): 5453-5472.

Lauritzen, Lotte, et al. "DHA Effects in Brain Development and Function." *Nutrients*. 2016 Jan; 8(1): 6.

Luchsinger, Jose, Tang Ming-Xin, Joshua Miller, et al. "Relation of Higher Folate Intake to Lower Risk of Alzheimer's Disease in the Elderly." *Archives of Neurology.* 2007; 64(1): 86-92.

Mayo Clinic. "Mediterranean Diet: A Heart-Healthy Eating Plan." Accessed November 30, 2018. https://www.mayoclinic.org/healthy-lifestyle/nutrition-and-healthy-eating/in-depth/mediterranean-diet/art-20047801.

Mayo Clinic. "Red Wine and Resveratrol: Good for Your Heart?" Accessed December 2, 2018. https://www.mayoclinic.org/diseases-conditions/heart-disease/in-depth/red-wine/art-20048281.

Mayo Clinic. "Water: Essential to Your Body." Accessed December 2, 2018. https://mayoclinic healthsystem.org/hometown-health/speaking-of-health/water-essential-to-your-body.

Mayo Clinic. "Water: How Much Should You Drink Every Day?" Accessed December 3, 2018. https://www.mayoclinic.org/healthy-lifestyle/nutrition-and-healthy-eating/in-depth/water/art-20044256.

McEvoy, C.T., H. Guyer, K.M. Langa, and K. Yaffe. "Neuroprotective Diets are Associated With Better Cognitive Function: The Health and Retirement Study." *Journal of the American Geriatrics Society.* 2017 Aug; 65(8): 1857-1862.

Michigan Medicine: The University of Michigan. "Avoiding Mercury in Fish." Accessed January 3, 2019. https://www.uofmhealth.org/health-library/tn6745spec.

Miller, M.G., D.A. Hamilton, J.A. Joseph, and B. Shukitt-Hale. "Dietary Blueberry Improves Cognition Among Older Adults in a Randomized, Double-Blind, Placebo-Controlled Trial." *European Journal of Nutrition.* 2018 Apr; 57(3): 1169-1180.

Mock, J. Thomas, Kiran Chaunhair, Akram Sidhu, and Nathalie Sumien. "The Influence of Vitamins E and C and Exercise on Brain Aging." *Experimental Gerontology.* 2017 Aug; 94: 69-72.

Morris, M.C. "The Role of Nutrition in Alzheimer's Disease: Epidemiological Evidence." *European Journal of Neurology.* 2009 Sep; 16(Suppl 1): 1-7.

Morris, M.C., D.A. Evans, J.L. Bienias, C.C. Tangney, and R.S. Wilson. "Vitamin E and Cognitive Decline in Older Persons." *Archives of Neurology.* 2002 Jul;59(7):1125-32.

Morris, M.C., et al. "Dietary Fats and the Risk of Incident Alzheimer's Disease." *Archives of Neurology.* 2003 Aug; 60(8): 1072.

Morris, M.C., D.A. Evans, C.C. Tangney, J.L. Bienias, and R.S. Wilson. "Associations of Vegetable and Fruit Consumption with Age-Related Cognitive Change." *Neurology.* 2006 Oct 24; 67(8): 1370-1376.

Morris, Martha Clare, Denis Evans, Julia Bienias, et al. "Consumption of Fish and N-3 Fatty Acids and Risk of Incident Alzheimer's Disease." *Archives of Neurology.* 2003;60(7):940-946.

Morris, Martha Clare, et al. "MIND Diet Slows Cognitive Decline with Aging." *Alzheimer's & Dementia.* 2016 Sep; 11(9): 1015-1022.

Morris, Martha Clare, Christy Tangney, Yamin Wang, Frank Sacks, David Bennett, and Aggarwal Neelum. "MIND Diet Associated with Reduced Incidence of Alzheimer's Disease." *Alzheimer's and Dementia.* 2015 September; 11(9): 1007-1014.

Morris, Martha Clare. *Diet for the Mind.* New York: Little, Brown and Company, 2017.

Muldoon, Matthew, Christopher Ryan, Jeffrey Yao, Sarah Conklin, and Stephen Manuck. "Long-Chain Omega-3 Fatty Acids and Optimization of Cognitive Performance." *Military Medicine*. 2014 Nov; 179(11 0): 95-105.

Mullan, K., et al. "Serum Concentrations of Vitamin E and Carotenoids are Altered in Alzheimer's Disease: A Case-Control Study." *Alzheimer's & Dementia*. 2017 Jul 19; 3(3): 432-439.

Nagamatsu, Lindsay, Todd Handy, C. Liang Hsu, Michelle Voss, and Teresa Liu-Ambrose. "Resistance Training Promotes Cognitive and Functional Brain Plasticity in Seniors with Probable Mild Cognitive Impairment: A 6-Month Randomized Controlled Trial." *Archives of Internal Medicine*. 2012 Apr; 172(8): 666-668.

Naqvi, Asghar, Brian Harty, Kenneth Mukamal, Anne Stoddard, Mara Vitolins, and Julie Dunn. "Monounsaturated, Trans, and Saturated Fatty Acids and Cognitive Decline in Women." *Journal of the American Geriatrics Society*. 2011 May; 59(5).

National Heart, Lung, and Blood Institute. "How Much Physical Activity Should Your Family Get?" Accessed December 3, 2018. https://www.nhlbi.nih.gov/health/educational/wecan/get-active /physical-activity-guidelines.htm.

National Institute of Mental Health. "5 Things You Should Know About Stress." Accessed December 1, 2018. https://www.nimh.nih.gov/health/publications/stress/index.shtml.

National Institute on Aging. "A Good Night's Sleep." Accessed December 1, 2018. https://www.nia.nih. gov/health/good-nights-sleep.

National Institute on Aging. "Alzheimer's Disease Genetics Fact Sheet." Accessed on November 23, 2018. https://www.nia.nih.gov/health/alzheimers-disease-genetics-fact-sheet

National Institute on Aging. "Preventing Alzheimer's Disease: What Do We Know?" Accessed on November 23, 2018. https://www.nia.nih.gov/health/preventing-alzheimers-disease -what-do-we-know.

National Institutes of Health. "Omega-3 Fatty Acids." Accessed November 26, 2018. https://ods .od.nih.gov/factsheets/Omega3FattyAcids-Consumer.

O'Brien, J., O. Okereke, E. Devore, B. Rosner, M. Breteler, and F. Grodstein. "Long-Term Intake of Nuts in Relation to Cognitive Function in Older Women." *Journal of Nutrition, Health and Aging*. 2014 May; 18(5): 496-502.

Oregon State University. "Flavonoids." Accessed November 26, 2018. https://lpi.oregonstate.edu /mic/dietary-factors/phytochemicals/flavonoids.

Panche, A.N., A.D. Diwan, and S.R. Chandra. "Flavonoids: an Overview." *Journal of Nutritional Science*. 2016; 5: 47.

Phillips, C. "Lifestyle Modulators of Neuroplasticity: How Physical Activity, Mental Engagement, and Diet Promote Cognitive Health During Aging." *Neural Plasticity*. June 2017.

Popkin, Barry, Kristen D'Anci, and Irwin Rosenberg. "Water, Hydration and Health." *Nutrition Reviews*. 2010 Aug; 68(8): 439-458.

Romagnolo, Donato. "Mediterranean Diet and Prevention of Chronic Diseases." *Nutrition Today*. 2017 Sep; 52(5) 208-22.

Seafood Health Facts: Making Smart Choices. "Omega-3 Content of Frequently Consumed Seafood Products." Accessed November 30, 2018. https://www.seafoodhealthfacts.org/seafood-nutrition /healthcare-professionals/omega-3-content-frequently-consumed-seafood-products.

Spencer, Jeremy. "Flavonoids and Brain Health: Multiple Effects Underpinned by Common Mechanisms." *Genes & Nutrition*. 2009; 4:136.

Steptoe, Andrew and Mika Kivimaki. "Stress and Cardiovascular Disease." *Nature Reviews Cardiology*. 2012; 9: 360-370.

Tangney, C.C., H. Li, Y. Wang, L. Barnes, J.A. Schneider, D.A. Bennett, and M.C. Morris. "Relation of DASH- and Mediterranean-Like Dietary Patterns to Cognitive Decline in Older Persons." *Neurology*. 2014 Oct; 83(16): 1410-6.

Toledo E., et al. "Effect of the Mediterranean Diet on Blood Pressure in the PREDIMED Trial: Results from a Randomized Controlled Trial." *BMC Medicine*. 2013 Sep 19; 11:207.

U.S. News & World Report. "What is the DASH Diet?" Accessed November 30, 2018. https://health.usnews.com/best-diet/dash-diet.

University of Michigan. "Vitamin B-Complex." Accessed November 21, 2018. https://www.uofm ealth.org/health-library/hn-2922005.

USDA Snap-Ed Connection. "Seasonal Produce Guide." Accessed December 7, 2018. https://snaped .fns.usda.gov/seasonal-produce-guide.

USDA. "Choose My Plate." Accessed December 5, 2018. https://www.choosemyplate.gov.

USDA. "Dietary Guidelines for Americans 2015-2020." Accessed December 7, 2018. https://www.choosemyplate.gov/dietary-guidelines.

Valls-Pedret, et al. "Polyphenol-Rich Foods in the Mediterranean Diet are Associated with Better Cognitive Function in Elderly Subjects at High Cardiovascular Risk." *Journal of Alzheimer's Disease*. 2012; 29: 773-782.

Vasanthi, Hannah, Royapuram Parameswari, Joel deLeiris, and Dipak Das. "Health Benefits of Wine and Alcohol from Neuroprotection to Heart Health." *Frontiers in Bioscience*. 2012 Jan; 4: 1505-1512.

Wang, Hui-Xin, Anita Karp, Bengt Winblad, and Laura Fratiglioni. "Late-Life Engagement in Social and Leisure Activities is Associated with a Decreased Risk of Dementia: A Longitudinal Study From The Kungsholmen Project." *American Journal of Epidemiology*. 2002 Jun; 155(12): 1081-1087.

WebMD. "The MIND Diet May Help Prevent Alzheimer's." Accessed November 21, 2018. https://www.webmd.com/alzheimers/features/mind-diet-alzheimers-disease#2.

Weiser, Michael, Christopher Butt, and M. Hasan Mohajeri. "Docosahexaenoic Acid and Cognition Throughout the Lifespan." *Nutrients*. 2016 Feb; 8(2): 99.

Wengreen H., et al. "Prospective Study of Dietary Approaches to Stop Hypertension- and Mediterranean-Style Dietary Patterns and Age-Related Cognitive Change: The Cache County Study on Memory, Health and Aging." *American Journal of Clinical Nutrition*. 2013 Nov; 98(5): 1263-71.

Wilson, R.S., et al. "Proneness to Psychological Distress is Associated with Risk of Alzheimer's Disease." *Neurology*. 2003 Dec; 61(11).

Wilson, R.S., P.A. Boyle, B.D. James, S.E. Leurgans, A.S. Buchman, and D.A. Bennett. "Negative Social Interactions and Risk of Mild Cognitive Impairment in Old Age." *Neuropsychology*. 2015 Jul; 29(4): 561-70.

Yuan, Changzheng, et al. "Long-Term Intake of Vegetables and Fruits and Subjective Cognitive Function in Med." *Neurology*. 2018 Nov.

Zabel, M., A. Nackenoff, W.M. Kirsch, F.E. Harrison, G. Perry, and M. Schrag. "Markers of Oxidative Damage to Lipids, Nucleic Acids and Proteins and Antioxidant Enzymes Activities in Alzheimer's Disease Brain: A Meta-Analysis in Human Pathological Specimens." *Free Radical Biology &Medicine*. 2018 Feb 1; 115: 351-360.

Index

Acknowledgments

To Ben, my feisty, adventurous, and witty husband, who is the most supportive person in my life. You've always encouraged me and indulged in my wild and crazy dreams, and I'll always be grateful for that. Without you, I wouldn't get to do what I love to do every single day.

To my parents, Jim and Jan, and sister, Jessie, who are my biggest cheerleaders. And my niece, Lacey, who I just know will love to cook when she's a bit older.

To my friends and colleagues who taught me cool things and encouraged me to be myself, do my own thing, and shoot for the stars. You know who you are.

To my high school science teacher, Mrs. Holman, who used to sing songs about photosynthesis. My mom swears you're the reason I fell in love with science.

To the Callisto publishing team, who took a chance on a new author and supported me through this journey. This experience has been a blessing.

To Dr. Martha Clare Morris, who authored the MIND diet, and to Dr. Morris and the Rush University Medical Center team, who conducted and published groundbreaking Alzheimer's and dementia research to support it. You made this book possible and are helping so many people. Keep up the amazing work.

And to everyone who follows The Gourmet RD, cooks my recipes, and shares them with the world. You're seriously the best.

About the Author

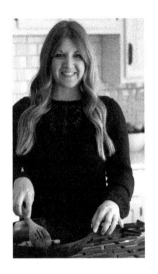

Julie Andrews, MS, RDN, CD, is a registered dietitian nutritionist and trained chef with a master's degree in human nutrition. She is the creator and owner of The Gourmet RD, where she is a food and nutrition consultant, cookbook author, recipe developer, food photographer, food and nutrition writer, and culinary media expert. She is regularly featured on television and in the media, where she shares nutrition expertise and showcases simple, wholesome, and delicious recipes from her blog, The-GourmetRD.com. Julie's greatest passion is helping others build confidence in the kitchen and inspiring them to cook for themselves, as she truly believes it's the ticket to better health and a more enjoyable life.

CPSIA information can be obtained
at www.ICGtesting.com
Printed in the USA
BVHW050142080519
547631BV00001BB/1

9 781641 524421